BODYWORK
SHIATSU

BODYWORK
SHIATSU

Bringing the Art of

Finger Pressure

to the

Massage Table

CARL DUBITSKY

HEALING ARTS PRESS
ONE PARK STREET
ROCHESTER, VERMONT 05767
WWW.GOTOIT.COM

Note to the reader: This book is intended as an informational guide. The remedies,
approaches, and techniques described herein are meant to supplement, and not to be a substitute
for, professional medical care or treatment. They should not be used to treat a serious ailment
without prior consultation with a qualified health-care professional. The author can be contacted
at HealthSprings Clinic, 4610 Arapahoe #2, Boulder, CO 80303, (303) 449-0800,
e-mail cdubi@mystical.net

LIBRARY OF CONGRESS CATALOGING-IN-PUBLICATION DATA

Dubitsky, Carl
Bodywork shiatsu: bringing the art of finger pressure to the
massage table/Carl Dubitsky.
p. cm.
Includes bibliographical references.
ISBN 0-89281-526-4
1. Acupressure. 2. Massage I. Title
RM723.A27D83 1997
615.8'22—dc20   89-20026
CIP
r96

Printed and bound in the United States

10 9 8 7 6 5 4 3 2 1

Text design by Dede Cummings
Text layout by Virginia L. Scott
Illustrations by Jennifer Veser
This book was typeset in Galliard with Anna and Univers as the display typefaces
Photographs of the table treatments by Lew Grothe feature Sharon Sager and Uma Basco
Photographs of the chair treatments by Isabelle Cozart feature Sharon Sager and the author
Photographs of the stances in chapter 9 feature Dennis Solem
The Deep Bodyworker massage table and the Portal Pro #2 massage chair shown in
the treatment photographs were provided by Oakworks, Inc.

Healing Arts Press is a division of Inner Traditions International
Distributed to the book trade in Canada by Publishers Group West (PGW), Toronto, Ontario
Distributed to the health food trade in Canada by Alive Books, Toronto and Vancouver
Distributed to the book trade in the United Kingdom by Deep Books, London
Distributed to the book trade in Australia by Millennium Books, Newtown, N. S. W.
Distributed to the book trade in New Zealand by Tandem Press, Auckland
Distributed to the book trade in South Africa by Alternative Books, Ferndale

This book is for my mother and my brother.

I OFFER THIS BOOK TO THE many teachers I have had in the various arts of hand healing, each of whom has added some vital aspect to my understanding of my craft. I offer this work to the thousands of clients who have not only provided me with the laboratory wherein I have mastered my skills, but have also given me constant inspiration and the experience of the true joy of service. They have taught me that "giving is a gift for the giver"! And finally, I offer this to all mankind with the profound hope that by learning to release each other's suffering, we may all begin the process of transcending the petty distinctions that keep us from experiencing the unconditional love that is our birthright.

I also offer my gratitude to the innumerable people who have helped, in large or small ways, over the years. Although there are too many to name individually, I give you all my humble thanks.

CONTENTS

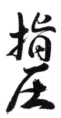

PART 4: FULL-BODY TREATMENT

FOREWORD

指圧

BODYWORK SHIATSU was originally conceived by the author as a workbook for his students. As such it is an extremely important addition to the literature in its specific field. Its thoroughness and precision provide the depth of concrete information that is missing from virtually all other shiatsu training manuals that I have seen. Especially helpful are the careful verbal descriptions that accompany the illustrations of pathways and treatment procedures. These are invaluable aids in accurately locating the meridians on the body. Their anatomical specificity dispels the ambiguity that plagues almost all graphic illustrations of the Oriental energy system.

But as excellent as it is in its genre, *BodyWork Shiatsu* is far more than just a training manual. It is a well-researched and thoughtful bridge between bodywork and modern medicine and between the mutually supportive truths of ancient and modern sciences. It is a significant exploration into the concrete anatomical, physiological, and neurological reasons why shiatsu in particular—and bodywork in general—can be such effective therapeutic tools.

Contrary to the biochemical models that currently dominate medical treatment, we are not just a collection of chemicals, tissues, and functional organs. We are also a collection of processes, habits, and developments, in active relationship with the forces within us and around us. We are delicately balanced ecosystems that are perpetually contending with such things as gravity, architectural (postural) stresses, fluid circulation, sensory input (or the lack of it), intake and diffusion of nutrients, and removal of waste products. Like all ecosystems, we must constantly keep up a dynamic motion, resolving acute crises and chronic tendencies before they permanently damage that balance. And the ways that we deal with these continually changing circumstances have just as much to do with our health and vitality as do genetic blueprints, physical traumas, and external disease agents.

It is in this broad context that the author grounds his discussion of the therapeutic effectiveness of bodywork. And it is in this context that the claims of its practitioners, both ancient and modern, begin to make perfect sense. Effective touch and the subjective impressions that guide it are not at all intuitive mumbo-jumbo; they are learnable skills with demonstrable, measurable results. Drawing on Dr. Hans Selye's descriptions of the general stress syndrome, Dr. Robert O. Becker's work with the subtle electrical currents coursing through the organism, modern research in biofeedback, and a wealth of currently accepted physiological data, this book makes a powerful case for an ancient medicine.

Such arguments are critically important to the development of health care at the present time. The practice of medicine is becoming dangerously dehumanized. Touching, examining, and providing physical comfort—elements that for centuries were a vital part of dealing with illness—have been drained away to a degree that would have shocked physicians only two generations ago. What we are now pleased to call "traditional" medicine is an outgrowth of a technology that did not exist the day before yesterday. While it does indeed work its miracles, there is absolutely no reason why we must discard older, still effective tools to do so. In fact, it is becoming universally acknowledged that many of the major killers and debilitators in our modern culture—cardiovascular disease, cancer, arthritis, respiratory diseases, and many immunological malfunctions—are directly related to emotional and physical stresses. And pharmaceuticals and surgery face insurmountable limitations in what they can do for these stress-induced conditions.

Styles of health care are of necessity changing rapidly in this country. Preventive medicine, the education of patients, and the active engagement of their own powers of self-regulation are developments that are going to revolutionize the field in a generation or two, just as surely as did penicillin, X-ray, and surgery.

BodyWork Shiatsu is a book that helps to put touch therapies squarely into the midst of these changes. At a time when our own technological hubris is forcing us to reexamine some of the more organic wisdoms of the ancients, and when we as a culture are looking with fascination at the spiritual traditions, economic successes, and sociological patterns of Japan and other countries in the East, perhaps we will come to recognize that the art of effective touch and the precise subjective impressions upon which it is based may well be one of the most valuable things we can borrow from them. Carl Dubitsky's work is certainly a step in this direction.

Deane Juhan
Mill Valley, California

PREFACE

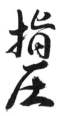

East or West: $E = mc^2$

At the dawn of the twentieth century Albert Einstein announced to the Western scientific world a radically new insight into the nature of reality. In his theory of relativity, he showed that energy and matter are not two different entities but complementary aspects of a single unified whole. This concept stunned the scientific community. It was so simple and yet foreign to mainstream scientific thought that it was said only eight people in the world understood what he was talking about. By the middle of this century, Western scientists had so well succeeded in integrating Einstein's insights that they were able to demonstrate the real-world applicability of these ideas with devastating impact.

At the dawn of time, the ancient Chinese scientist/philosophers understood the relative nature of reality, and they developed their entire medical science around that understanding. Today, Western medicine is just beginning to reflect that earth-shaking change in our worldview.

In the field of health care, the Western scientific approach has led to a remarkable understanding of the structure of the human bodymind through rigorous differentiation. The Eastern cultural approach, on the other hand, has led to a very keen and utilitarian understanding of pattern and function based on the perceived unity of that same bodymind.

These two disparate views—of flowing patterns or discrete structures—both describing the real world, allow for remarkably evolved medical paradigms and lead to truly awesome medical accomplishments. We can use either viewpoint as a basis for analyzing disease in the human body and arrive at radically different descriptions of identical conditions. Both provide useful insights into the nature of human suffering as well as the means to alleviate it.

In this book we will examine the art-science of BodyWork Shiatsu from both perspectives. Experience has taught me that in some circumstances energetic manipulation, treatment designed to balance energy, is most effective, while in other circumstances structural bodywork, treatment intended to alter physical structure, is more effective.

What I find amazing is that in both cases my hands appear to be doing the same things. Only the perceptual framework and intention, the conceptual paradigm, differs.

We will begin with an overview of traditional Chinese medicine and then review the subject in terms of Western anatomy and physiology. Both approaches yield remarkable insights. We will conclude with a step-by-step description of how to give a full BodyWork Shiatsu session on a massage table as well as an introductory treatment designed for a seated client.

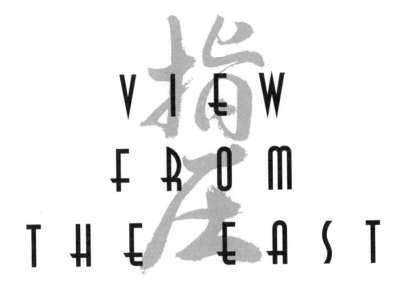

PART 1

VIEW FROM THE EAST

CHAPTER 1

ORIGINS AND OBJECTIVES OF BODYWORK SHIATSU

ORIENTAL MEDICINE in general, and its manipulative procedures in particular, represent one of humankind's most evolved forms of preventive medicine. BodyWork Shiatsu is the integration of several different forms of Japanese shiatsu and anma, Chinese tuina, and Western osteopathic, physiotherapeutic, and therapeutic massage and bodywork techniques that are woven together according to the needs of the client at each session. It is recognized as a form of both shiatsu/anma and integrative/eclectic shiatsu as described below.

Shi means finger, *atsu* means pressure. The Japanese Ministry of Health and Welfare defines shiatsu therapy as "a form of manipulation administered by the thumbs, fingers, and palms, without the use of any instrument, mechanical or otherwise, to apply pressure to the human skin, correct internal malfunctioning, promote and maintain health and treat specific diseases."[1] The ministry lists over two hundred medical problems for which shiatsu is a primary treatment modality.[2]

Anma represents the ancient lineage of traditional Oriental hand-healing. *An* means press, and *ma* means stroke. Derived from the Chinese *anmo*, which was brought to Japan in the sixth century C.E., anma treatment is a fluid massage form that consists of applying pressure, stroking, and other forms of manipulation to the energetic points and pathways that are identified in Oriental medicine, as well as all of the other soft tissues of the body. Anma has been developed in countless schools and families in both China and Japan, as well as all other countries of southeast Asia. The number of different hands-on techniques that fall under the category of anma massage is vast, as are the number of diagnostic and therapeutic approaches employed. Properly speaking, all hand therapies that assess and treat the energetic system are part of the anma lineage.

In the fall of 1989 the American Oriental Bodywork Therapy Association (AOBTA) adopted the following definition of Oriental bodywork, which is inclusive of shiatsu/anma therapy.

Oriental Bodywork Therapy: The treatment of the human body, including the electromagnetic or energetic field which surrounds, infuses, and brings that body to life, by pressure and/or manipulation. This approach is based upon traditional Oriental medical principles for assessing and evaluating the energetic system, and traditional Oriental techniques and treatment strategies to primarily affect and balance the energetic system, for the purpose of treating the human body, emotions, mind, energy field, and spirit for the promotion, maintenance, and restoration of health.

When based on appropriate education, adjunctive modalities within the scope of Oriental Bodywork Therapy are non-invasive. They include, but are not limited to, pressure devices, application of hot and cold, external application of herbal or chemical preparations, electromagnetic treatment modalities, and education regarding appropriate principles of diet and therapeutic exercises.[3]

It is my experience that, regardless of its focus, Oriental bodywork affects not only the energetic system but also the superficial and deep tissues, and the fascial, myofascial, neuromuscular, musculoskeletal, circulatory, lymphatic, respiratory, digestive, eliminative, and craniosacral systems.[4] These additional realms that Oriental bodywork influences will be further discussed in chapter 6.

HISTORY OF ORIENTAL BODYWORK THERAPY

The origins of Oriental bodywork stretch back into the mists of Chinese antiquity. In the oldest written medical text still in existence, the *Huang Di Nei Jing Su Wen* (translated into English as *The Yellow Emperor's Classic of Internal Medicine*), dated from the first century B.C.E., the mythical first emperor of China, Huang Di, asks his premier physician, Qi Bo, to describe the role of bodywork in Oriental medicine. The great healer replied:

In the spring and autumn, when food is plentiful and humans tend to become lazy and slothful, finger pressure is used to increase digestive fire and restore vigor.[5]

Northern and southern China were unified during the Qin dynasty in the third century B.C.E. Oriental bodywork was called *moshou* (hand rubbing) at that time. By the fifth century C.E., the science of Oriental bodywork therapy had evolved to such a level that a doctoral degree was created at the Imperial College of Medicine in Xian, the ancient capital of the Tang dynasty. Every Chinese medical physician was required to master moshou in order to help them develop the refined palpation skills necessary for diagnostics and for the competent practice of acupuncture. Oriental bodywork therapy has been known as *anmo* (press and stroke) since the Han dynasty (206 B.C.E.–220 C.E.), and *tuina* (lift and grasp) since the Ming dynasty (1368–1664 C.E.). It has been a distinct medical specialty in every successive dynasty in China up to the present day, with medical schools and hospitals devoted exclusively to its practice, and departments of Oriental bodywork in every general medical school and hospital in the country.[6]

Chinese medicine was brought to Japan by the Buddhist priest Gan Jin Osho during the Nara Jidai Tempyo period, in the sixth century C.E. (the date traditionally given is 552 C.E.[7]), when he accompanied the entourage of the trade embassy from the imperial Chinese court and taught Japanese healers the medicine of imperial China. The manipulative portions of *kampo* (Chinese medicine) have always appealed to the Japanese temperament, as a result of which Oriental bodywork, acupuncture, moxibustion, and palpatory diagnosis have been developed by the Japanese to an extraordinary degree.

The physical therapies reached a peak in Japan during the Edo period (1603–1867). During this period, just as in China thousands of years earlier, every physician was required to master Oriental bodywork before being allowed to diagnose or use needles.

The major force in the development of Japanese medicine during this period was Waichi Sugiyama (1614–1694). Blind from the age of one, Sugiyama left his home in Kyoto and went to Edo (Tokyo) as a teenager, in hopes of studying anma massage under Ryomei Irie, the foremost master of Oriental medicine then practicing in Japan. After a short period of apprenticeship Irie decided that Sugiyama was too dull a student and dismissed him, sending him back home to Kyoto.

On the journey home Sugiyama made a pilgrimage to the shrine of the goddess Benten (Hindu: Saraswati), on the Isle of Enoshima, near Kamakura. Fasting and praying for seven days at the feet of the goddess, Sugiyama had a vision in which the goddess told him to return to Edo, and handed him the needle insertion tube with which he revolutionized Japanese acupuncture.

Later in his life Sugiyama was brought to treat the fifth Tokugawa shogun, Lord Tsunayoshi. Tsunayoshi was suffering from a painful abdominal illness that none of the court physicians had been able to cure. When Sugiyama was able to rapidly return the shogun to good health, Lord Tsunayoshi returned the favor by naming Sugiyama superintendent of blind people and helping him found forty-five medical schools for blind people all over Japan, earning him the sobriquet "the father of Japanese acupuncture and bodywork."[8]

European medicine was introduced to the Japanese by commercial traders around the turn of the nineteenth century, and because of its cultural cachet, surgical methods, and efficacy in treating infectious diseases, it was adopted by the aristocracy, who forbade the teaching or use of the native Oriental therapies. During the Meiji dynasty (1868–1912), a simplified form of traditional anma massage was taught to all blind persons by imperial decree, in order to enable them to earn their livelihood. European massage was also incorporated into anma schooling. Practitioners were called "anma shampooers." Because so much of the diagnostic power of koho (ancient technique) anma was lost in the simplified form, anma massage degenerated into a pleasurable indulgence for the rich and powerful.

In 1911 the first law regulating the practice of acupuncture, moxibustion, and anma massage was introduced. This forced practitioners of the "ancient way" healing therapies to create new names for their work in order to avoid these licensing laws.[9]

In 1919 Tamai Tempaku published a book entitled Shiatsu Ho (Finger-pressure therapy). Tamai had studied and practiced koho anma for many years and had studied the Chinese acupoint system. He specialized in ampuku, abdominal massage, which had originally come from China but was further developed and extensively practiced in Japan. He studied the textbook Ampuku Zukai (Diagrams of hara treatment) by Ota Heisai, which became the standard text for Oriental abdominal therapy.[10] Tamai practiced and taught do-in (dao yin), Oriental breathing practices and physical exercises to circulate vital energy and help to integrate the bodymind. He also thoroughly studied Western anatomy and physiology and European massage.

Although Tamai had previously published a book, Shiatsu Ryoho (Finger pressure way of healing) in 1915, the attention of the therapeutic bodywork community did not focus on his work until Shiatsu Ho was released. This book described a system that integrated koho anma, ampuku, acupoint therapy, do-in, and Western anatomy and physiology. In it Tamai described treatments for a variety of Western ailments using traditional Oriental bodywork techniques, and he integrated traditional spiritual wisdom with his modern medicine. In the preface he wrote:

> People must have high spiritual development to do shiatsu, because healing disease is not only by fingertip pressure. You have to have spiritual power to do healing by hand.[11]

Tamai Tempaku's application of Western anatomical and physiological information to his treatment system was revolutionary. Tossed into the ferment that was taking place in the Japanese therapeutic community because of the onslaught of a host of poorly trained anma practitioners and the input of European medicine, his ideas stimulated a large group of traditional practitioners to pursue similar lines of inquiry. Katsusuke Serizawa and Tokujiro Namikoshi, as well as the mother of Shizuto Masunaga, were among his students.

In 1925 the Shiatsu Therapists Association was formed in order to distinguish practitioners of Oriental bodywork therapy from the anma shampooers practicing massage for general relaxation. Also in 1925 Takichi Tsukuba published *Akahon* (Red book: the secret of true treatment). This one-volume compendium of the works of Tamai Tempaku became the handbook for many students of Japanese bodywork therapies. Practitioners followed various lines of inquiry, and eventually a number of different bodywork therapies were developed based on Tamai's earlier work. Three of these student-practitioners founded schools that still exert a major influence on the study and practice of shiatsu/anma today: Serizawa Sensei, Masunaga Sensei, and Tokujiro Namikoshi Sensei.

After studying with Tempaku, Serizawa Sensei went on to study physical therapy at the Tokyo School of Education for the Blind, completing the instructors' course in 1938. He began physiological research at Tokyo University in 1951 and in 1955 became a research fellow at the Tokyo University School of Medicine with Professor Yoshio Oshima. He was awarded a Doctor of Medicine degree in 1961 for his research into the *tsubo* (acupoint) system. Using the electrometric measuring devices just becoming available to the Japanese medical community, he was able to prove beyond any doubt the actual physical existence of the acupoint system of Oriental medical theory. Serizawa Sensei developed the Oriental bodywork technique called tsubo therapy and in 1976 published the landmark book *Tsubo: Vital Points for Oriental Therapy*.

Masunaga Sensei began his study of shiatsu following his graduation from Kyoto University with a degree in psychology. After studying and teaching at the Nippon Shiatsu Institute for ten years, Masunaga began to pursue his own theories on the energetic structure of the human body. Based upon his clinical research, Masunaga created a unique synthesis of traditional Oriental theory and personal discovery which he called Zen shiatsu. Where Serizawa focused on the acupoints, Masunaga developed a system based on treating the meridian system of the body. He also developed a complex system for abdominal and back diagnosis and an extended set of meridians unique to his style. Masunaga published *Zen Shiatsu* in 1977.

The most famous practitioner, and the man most responsible for the recognition shiatsu has achieved both in Japan and worldwide, was Tokujiro Namikoshi. Gifted as a healer since childhood, Namikoshi Sensei first began developing his remarkable talents by treating his mother's rheumatism. After studying koho anma and European massage, he founded the Clinic of Appaku Ho (the pressure way) on Hokkaido in 1925. The clinic name was soon changed to the Shiatsu Institute of Therapy in response to the tremendous popular acceptance of the term *shiatsu* taking place on the mainland.

In 1933 Namikoshi moved to Tokyo, where he encountered tremendous difficulty in establishing himself. Finally, in 1939, he cured a well-known Hokkaido politician, Ishmaru Gohay, of a chronic and very painful back problem; Gohay rewarded him with $10,000 in Juman yen, a fortune in those days. Gohay also insured Namikoshi Sensei's hands. These events encouraged Namikoshi to open the Nippon Shiatsu Institute in Tokyo in 1940. Namikoshi then began petitioning to have shiatsu recognized separately from anma massage.

In his attempt to distance his system from the old-fashioned, prescientific connotations of anma massage, Namikoshi Sensei eliminated all references to traditional Oriental medical concepts from his therapy. He described the effects of his work in Western scientific medical terms, effectively creating a system that we would today call neuromuscular massage.[12]

In the post–World War II reorganization of all aspects of Japanese life that took place under the occupation forces of the Allied armies, *harikyu shiatsu*, as Japanese medicine is termed, was at first outlawed,[13] only to be reinstated due to the enormous outcry of the Japanese people. Then in 1953 a remarkable event took place, one that was destined to change the course of shiatsu's history. After being married in the United States, Joe DiMaggio and Marilyn Monroe went to Japan for their honeymoon. While in Tokyo Marilyn became deathly ill and failed to respond to the Western medical treatment she received. As a last resort Namikoshi Sensei was called in; he went to their hotel every day for a week to treat her. The remarkable recovery of the famous movie star became known all over Japan. Finally, in 1954 shiatsu was officially recognized by the Japanese government, albeit as a form of anma massage.

In 1955 the federal government took over the task of setting medical standards from the various local prefectures. Rigid qualifications, including three years of medical school and two years of residency, were required of all Oriental medical physicians before they were allowed to sit for a federal licensing examination. Bodywork licensure required two years of schooling. In 1964 shiatsu was finally recognized as a distinct speciality by the Japanese government.

Today shiatsu/anma is made available to the Japanese work force free of charge by all major industries because of the incredible decrease in time lost from the job by workers who receive regular preventive therapy. A more general form of shiatsu/anma is practiced in most households, both for its relaxing and invigorating qualities as well as for the tremendous closeness it brings to family members who care for each other with this oldest and most basic form of loving health care.

SHIATSU IN AMERICA

In 1950 Toshiko Phipps was the first qualified Japanese shiatsu therapist to begin teaching in America. In 1953 Toru Namikoshi, the son of Tokujiro Namikoshi, came to the United States and began teaching shiatsu at Palmer Chiropractic College in Ohio. The other teachers that Namikoshi Sensei sent to North America to continue to teach his method, Yukiko Irwin in the United States and Tetsu Saito in Canada, exclusively taught Namikoshi's neuromuscular approach to Oriental bodywork. Perhaps in an unconscious attempt to present a scientific face to Westerners, many teachers of other lineages who came to America also called their techniques shiatsu therapy.

There has been a fair amount of bickering over who originated the term *shiatsu therapy*. In 1965 Okura Sadakatsu wrote a series of articles entitled "Nippon No Ryo Jutsu" (Healing therapies of Japan) for the newspaper *Zen Ryo Shinbum*. He thoroughly researched the origins of shiatsu therapy and reported that Tamai Tempaku was clearly the founder of the shiatsu school of bodywork.

American students, concerned about rediscovering the basic life force that Western medicine had long ago discarded, proceeded to integrate, under the name *shiatsu*, all of the various hand techniques and energetic theories originally derived from koho anma, thus creating an American shiatsu/anma integration that I believe would be acceptable to Tamai Tempaku as well as to the ancient Chinese adepts. This reintegration was first introduced in America by Dr. DoAnn T. Kaneko.

Traditional anma massage, as taught by Dr. Kaneko, consists of seven basic techniques: pressing and stroking, grasping and kneading, strengthening, compression, vibration, tapotement, and hand music. Derived from Chinese anmo, anma massage is based on the energetic system of traditional Chinese medicine (TCM) and combines meridian massage and soft-tissue manipulation with the use of the acupoint system. Ancient and modern techniques of abdominal treatment (ampuku) are also incorporated. Evaluation is based on the Four Examinations: Looking, Asking, Smelling/Listening, and Touching. Findings are assessed according to the Eight Principles, and advanced treatments are based on the conditions found at the time of each treatment.

Shiatsu therapy, utilizing the style of Serizawa Sensei, is incorporated into this approach to treatment, adding direct compression of the nerve points, spinal correction, and active and passive exercises. Several basic forms emphasize either anma massage or shiatsu therapy as appropriate. Treatment is given in prone, supine, and side-lying positions, as well as in the seated position, using fingers, palms, elbows, and knees.

Combining traditional techniques of Oriental manipulation (koho anma) and abdominal therapy (ampuku) with modern Japanese shiatsu therapy, integrative/eclectic shiatsu also draws deeply from modern Western techniques of therapeutic sports massage and bodywork, including joint mobilization. While focusing on the meridian and acupoint systems of TCM, when appropriate, integrative/eclectic shiatsu treatment targets the neuromuscular, myofascial, musculoskeletal, craniosacral, visceral, lymphatic, venous, and neurological systems of Western medicine. Using the traditional Oriental diagnostic methods of Looking, Asking, Smelling/Listening, and Touching, patients are evaluated according to the Eight Principles, and appropriate treatments—using Eastern, Western, or combined techniques—are employed. Working both internally and externally, breathing, diet, herbs, exercise, and liniments are used as appropriate. Although primarily intended as preventive health care, integrative/eclectic shiatsu is extremely effective in treating all of the energetic, functional, organic, or soft-tissue diseases that are within the range of Oriental bodywork therapy.

The beginning level of practice taught in this book is called *sugi momi* (meridian treatment) by the Japanese.* The acupoints, called tsubo (hole or

*In this book I will use the term *meridian* to refer to the Organ-related energy conduits that connect the series of points related to each Organ on the surface of the body as well as to the deep course of each pathway that connects internally to its related Organ. I will refer to the pathways that connect meridians to meridians, or Organs to Organs, as well as the system that connects the meridians to all of the superficial tissues, as *channels*. I refer to the eight Extraordinary Pathways as well as the containers of Blood circulation as *vessels*. I will use the term *pathway* as a generic referent for all of these different aspects of the energetic system.

well) in Japanese, are the same for all systems of Oriental medicine. The Chinese discovered the acupoint and pathway systems by observation over the course of several thousand years. Over millennia a long succession of astute and observant practitioners noticed specific sequences of points and pathways on the surface of the body that became sensitive in reaction to the presence of internal organ dysfunction. Further, it was found that a variety of different manipulative techniques applied to the acupoints and meridians benefited the functioning of the organs associated with them.[14]

Certain of the acupoints correspond to the major trigger or reflex points that Western medicine now recognizes. Trigger points are the specific focus of muscular or myofascial disturbances. Reflex points are the superficial reflection of the conditions of the internal organs. McBurney's reflex point, in the lower right quadrant of the abdomen, becomes so sore in the presence of an inflamed appendix that it cannot be overlooked. The same is true for the pain that radiates from the armpit to the tip of the pinky finger during an attack of angina pectoris. This path of referred pain follows the Heart Meridian exactly. Refined and concentrated palpatory exploration of the body has revealed a host of sensitive reflex points associated with specific patterns of imbalance.

The kind of stimulus applied to the acupoints and meridians is a major determinant of the effect generated, although the way in which the stimulus is applied is also critical to the outcome. In general, needles are the most effective way to lower the energy in a specific region, while the application of heat, via moxibustion,[15] most effectively adds energy. The use of the hands forms a middle ground, allowing for tonification (addition) or sedation (subtraction) of vital energy as necessary. However, needles can also add, or moxa subtract, energy according to the technique used and the situation being treated. As in all aspects of Oriental medicine, everything is relative.

By applying hands-on techniques in accordance with a subtle and very sophisticated understanding of the bio-electromagnetic relationship between the surface of the body and its internal workings, Oriental bodywork helps to create and maintain the free and balanced flow of vital energy necessary for perfect health. Oriental bodywork is not only effective in correcting the energy imbalances that underlie a myriad of conditions, it is also the basis of a preventive health-care system that has, for thousands of years, helped its adherents maintain a dynamic state of vital health.

LEVELS OF TREATMENT

Oriental hand-healing techniques can be practiced at three levels: relaxation-level, or basic, Oriental bodywork; remedial-level, or intermediate, Oriental bodywork; and wholistic-level, or advanced, Oriental bodywork. Although many of the same techniques are used at every level, the training, experience, and skill required to effect specific changes increases dramatically with each progression.[16]

Relaxation-Level Oriental Bodywork
Relaxation-level Oriental bodywork, such as the BodyWork Shiatsu treatment taught in this text, is a full-body, pathway-oriented form of treatment primarily employed for general relaxation, increased vitality, and pure pleasure. Although vastly more effective, relaxation-level Oriental bodywork is comparable to Swedish massage in the context within which it is applied. Facilities throughout the Orient, including centers in all major industries, have Oriental bodywork practitioners set up to offer a shower, a sauna (to cleanse the skin), a heated futon (upon which to rest), and

a full-body, pathway-level treatment. No specific evaluation is involved; training is limited to learning the course and direction of the pathways and the appropriate hand and foot techniques for general stimulation. Because Oriental practitioners are frequently small in stature, much of this therapy is applied by the feet in order to generate adequate pressure. (Most American practitioners do not need to use their feet.)

Although not targeted toward curing specific conditions, the application of this level of treatment can re-create the free-flowing energy balance essential to true health. Relaxation-level Oriental bodywork lends itself well to a preventive health-care program designed to inhibit organic degeneration that leads to what we recognize as disease.

An American concept for marketing this level of treatment, called on-site massage, offers mini-treatments to clients seated in a chair at their place of work. These sessions require only fifteen minutes and are performed with the client fully clothed. Although much less comprehensive than a full-body treatment, the relaxing effects created by this sort of treatment, considering the time spent, is extraordinary. This nonthreatening introduction to Oriental bodywork is encouraging many people to further explore Oriental bodywork therapies. The promotional practice of on-site massage has always provided me with a full clientele within a very short time. This form is fully discussed in the treatment section (part 4).

Remedial-Level Oriental Bodywork

The second level of Oriental bodywork therapy focuses on the remediation of specific problems, including sprains or strains, postoperative or post-traumatic adhesions, restricted range of motion, and pathway-mediated muscular imbalances, as well as meridian and organ disorders, headaches, toothaches, menstrual disorders, digestive difficul-

ties, joint stiffness, certain sleep disorders, and general malaise. In addition to the study of the meridians, which is required for relaxation-level practice, the following skills are needed: a thorough grounding in the acupoint system, a knowledge of musculoskeletal anatomy, a complete understanding of the energetic anatomy of the meridian and channel systems, training in a variety of stimulative and sedative manipulation techniques, and memorization of various formulae for treating specific problems.

A level of evaluative skill able to assess the conditions presented for treatment, including the ability to differentiate meridian imbalances from organic problems; the ability to choose the correct Organ/meridian system(s) for treatment; and the knowledge of proper treatment protocol is necessary for this level of practice.

Wholistic-Level Oriental Bodywork

Orthodox Western medical culture lacks even the most rudimentary understanding of the most advanced level of Oriental bodywork therapy, however, the manipulative approaches to osteopathic medicine recognize preventive wholistic health care. To function at the primary health-care level, all practitioners must master the full panoply of diagnostic techniques and understand Oriental medical theory in all its intricate complexity. While primarily focused on manipulative therapies, the practitioner must be fully conversant with all aspects of Oriental medicine, including the use of needles, moxibustion, cupping, diet, herbs, exercise, breathing, and meditation. While superficially similar in appearance to the meridian-level practice, functioning at the wholistic level requires an ability to assess specific imbalances *before* they become symptomatic.

There is a story, perhaps anecdotal in nature, that in ancient China the physician would travel among his constituency evaluating each patient. He gave each patient the necessary Oriental bodywork, acupuncture, and moxibustion treatments; as well, he prescribed appropriate dietary, herbal, meditative, and breathing exercises to achieve and maintain perfect health. For this service he was wined and dined, and paid a pretty penny.

However, should disease occur in spite of patient compliance with his prescriptions, he was then required to stay and treat that patient at his own expense. Although subtle in nature, Oriental diagnosis is very exact; a competent doctor was expected to be able to detect and correct imbalanced energy function long before it manifested as physical degeneration.

THE YOGA OF BODYWORK SHIATSU

The domain of the Great Healer—the most refined and subtle practitioner of Oriental medicine—lies in recognizing and treating disease states before they manifest on the physical plane, requiring successful treatment of imbalanced conditions before symptoms ever develop. Herein lies the genius of Chinese medical theory. Remediation of actual disease was the work of second-class physicians at best.

At the heart of successful preventive health care is the practitioner's awareness and well-being. The art of healing requires an ability on the part of the practitioner to extend beyond the normal limits of self-concern in order to become one with the person being healed. Healing involves the ability to act as a focus of manifestation for the self-transcendent universal energy that is the true source of well-being. It requires the therapist to stand in a place of non-doing and non-knowing, and from that expansive place garner an intuitive understanding of right action that, when acted upon, can sever the knot of suffering. It is this very striving to become a pure vessel of the healing grace that leads us ever closer to the consciousness of unconditional love; it transforms the act of healing others into the act of healing self.

Recognizing and opening into this universal energy is at the heart of traditional Oriental medical training, making BodyWork Shiatsu, in its essence, a self-transformative discipline. All diagnostic techniques or treatment methods aside, BodyWork Shiatsu is primarily an opportunity for work on oneself. Lao Zi, the ancient Chinese sage and author of the *Dao De Jing*, points to the need for this essential process of self-development. Regarding the establishment of a concentrated center from which to function as a healer, he says:

> The five colors make a person's eyes blind.
> The five tones make a person's ears deaf.
> The five tastes make a person's mouth with
>   no sense of taste.
> Riding and hunting make a person's heart
>   crazy like a beast.
> Something which is hard to obtain disturbs
>   his path.
> Therefore the Chinese Sage [the Great
>   Healer] becomes the Hara [the abdomen].
> There he puts his consciousness.
> He doesn't become his eyes [foster identification with the senses].
> Therefore, throw away the one, and pick up
>   the other.[17]

Developing a well-tuned proprioceptive* sense is requisite to learning to allow the universal

---

* *Taber's Medical Dictionary* defines proprioception as "The awareness of posture, movement, and changes in equilibrium, and the knowledge of position, weight, and resistance of objects in relation to the body." Proprioceptive sense is defined as "The correlation of unconscious sensations from the skin and joints that allows conscious appreciation of the position of the body." Please see the section on proprioception in chapter 7 for a thorough discussion of this aspect of our sensorium, and the impact that concentrated focus on it has on consciousness.

healing energy to work through you. The proprioceptors are normally an aspect of the involuntary nervous system, and they are responsible for both detecting subtle body changes and guiding delicate, refined movement. Due to both the subtle nature of proprioceptive feedback and our Western cultural conditioning that demands gross verification of reality, information from this portion of the neural network usually flows outside the boundaries of our everyday, egoic consciousness. The steady proprioceptive focus required for the practice of BodyWork Shiatsu naturally leads to an ever wider and less self-centered state of awareness, allowing for the conscious integration of subtle thoughts, feelings, sensations, images, and intuitions. The constant attunement at the proprioceptive level required in receiving, processing, and transmitting information between client and practitioner ultimately transforms the act of giving a BodyWork Shiatsu treatment into the stillness of meditation.

In persistently striving to become more internally aware, better able to share with your client, in touch and in words, the universal knowledge that he or she needs to hear and feel in order to come into the balance of true health, a therapist must drop back and so invite spontaneous communication with the space of perfection inside us all. Treatment technique pales before the self-effulgent radiance of the inner Self, the realm of the Great Healer.

The information and techniques that follow provide a mere framework around which this communication may take place. We must learn the letters and words of this healing language, it is true. But we must, first and last, strive to become that instrument through which the Great Healer may clearly speak.

Purity of intention, selfless service, attention to detail, hard work, a great deal of study, good health habits, and above all the desire to nurture all beings: these are the qualities that lead to the mastery of BodyWork Shiatsu. This pathway leads to wholeness. May all who are sincerely interested reach this goal.

CHAPTER 2

ORIENTAL COSMOLOGY

THROUGHOUT HISTORY SCIENTISTS have sought a comprehensive description of the nature of reality. In the twentieth century that search has manifested in the physicists' quest for a unified field theory as a physical description of reality. The Western bias toward left-brained, objective proof, and the tendency to distinguish between the physical and mental aspects of reality, have confined proof of the concept of the unified field theory to the instrumentation of the scientific laboratory.

Culturally biased toward the right-brained, subtle, experiential information that is able to be received by the centered mind, the Eastern sages never made the distinction between mind and matter. Consequently, in the East, physical medicine and spiritual truth were founded on the same understanding of the nature of reality. Because the basic instrument of scientific research was the silent, concentrated mind, the Chinese description of the physical universe proceeded from the subtle to the gross. Conversely, Western science moves from the grossly perceptible to the ever more invisible.

The most esoteric descriptions of reality made by today's subatomic-particle physicists are indistinguishable from the philosophic writings of Chinese sages three thousand years ago.[1] Laboratory investigations have led modern physicists to define the basic stuff of subatomic structure as a ceaselessly transforming flux of infinite variety—particles changing into antiparticles, positive becoming negative, all able to be described equally as matter or energy, moving forward in time or backward. In fact, at the finest level perceivable with our most advanced instrumentation, we can tell either *what* a particle is, or *where* it is, but never both. The very act of observation alters what we see, leaving us with a mystical soup of indescribable complexity, endlessly dancing to a rhythm that beggars our imagination.

FORMLESSNESS

The Oriental cosmology began with that which cannot be described. The ancient sage Lao Zi said,

"He who knows cannot say, and he who says, does not know,"[2] for ultimate reality is the very substrate of the mind. The act of fixing it in words denies the ineffable truth of what it is or is not. Called the Dao (the Void or the Way), it corresponds to what the Christian world calls God Transcendent. It is that nameless, formless, silent emptiness within which play the endless interlocking rings of increasingly more concrete manifestation. Rather than describe it in dead and static words, the Eastern sages did so with a living symbol which, by its very nature, leads the mind to an appreciation of the ceaselessly transmogrifying nature of the Dao.

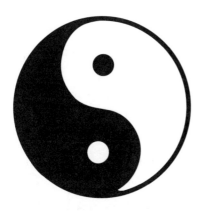

Fig. 2.1. The Dao (Ultimate Reality)

In their observations of the natural processes of manifestation from ultimate formlessness into form, the Eastern masters noticed two related concepts that were always operative. They termed these fundamental principles *the law of change* and *the law of complementarity*. They noticed that in the world nothing ever remains the same—everything is engaged in a constant state of change, cycling from one form to another and from one phase to another. They further noticed that these changes followed a cyclical pattern, swelling to fullness in one quality and then suddenly transforming into the comple-

mentary quality. Because they saw reality as a ceaseless process rather than a static condition or object, the Eastern symbol for reality circles endlessly. It does not increase infinitely in a linear direction; rather, the unmanifest potential for other aspects of its nature is always retained in any one expression of reality. Thus, at the maximum of one quality of its nature, manifest creation still contains the seed of its complement, and at the moment of greatest fullness it begins transforming into this complementary quality. Hence darkness does not infinitely increase, getting ever darker, but rather the peak of night is simultaneously the beginning of dawn; the longest day of summer is in fact the herald for the birth of winter's night.

YIN AND YANG

This cyclical interplay of complementary opposites was named Yin and Yang. The sages found this understanding of complementary opposition could be applied to everything in the universe—Heaven and Earth, masculine and feminine, light and dark, hot and cold, hard and soft, inside and outside—and that this process of division into polar opposites could be extended to include all aspects of known reality. The *Su Wen* (Simple questions) states:

> Yin and Yang can be divided down to ten, and then further down to one hundred, to a thousand, to ten thousand, and to a number so great it defies calculation: yet in essence all these are but one.[3]

They perceived these reciprocal polarities as totally interdependent: the very existence of one pole of the duality was only manifest because of its complement. It was said:

> Yang has its root in Yin; Yin has its root in Yang.

Without Yin, Yang cannot arise; without
    Yang, Yin cannot be born.
Yin alone cannot arise; Yang alone cannot
    grow.
Yin and Yang are divisible, but not
    separable.[4]

The Eastern sages observed Yin and Yang to be in a state of reciprocal equilibrium, constantly acting upon each other in order to maintain a harmonious balance. If one quality increases, the complement proportionally decreases. Each applies a constant counterbalancing pressure on the other, resisting a shift to imbalance in either direction. As we will see, this tendency toward maintaining equilibrium has important implications in the creation and maintenance of health and the remediation of disease.

THE ELEMENTS

Nothing is ever totally Yang or Yin, positive or negative. All things that we can sense are rather elementary manifestations of this interplay of opposites, and so, within the categories of Yin and Yang, we can further divide manifestation into its basic elemental forms—not the elements of the chemist's periodic table, but the solid, liquid, gaseous, fiery, and etheric nature of all things that can be seen and touched and tasted.

However, even this division is a mental abstraction, for the things of this world are never in a purely elemental form. The rarest vacuum (our modern scientific version of the ether) is still filled with stray atoms and their particles; the purest water has its parts per million of this or that impurity. Reality, at the level that our senses can perceive, is always an admixture of the ideal elements of theoretical conception.

THE TEN THOUSAND THINGS

The Chinese sages named the level of reality that is perceptible to our senses the Ten Thousand Things. They used the intersecting qualities of Yin and Yang and the subsequent five elementary transformations to form a descriptive picture that allowed for a workable description of manifest nature. This enabled the Oriental physician to successfully confront the apparently endless complexity of the human body.

HEAVENLY YANG/ EARTHLY YIN

In their development of the Five Element theory, the Chinese elaborated upon the interrelationships of the overlapping spheres of Yin and Yang, and delineated the effects of these interrelationships upon the Sphere of the Human. To the Chinese mind, macroscopic phenomena—events beyond the scope of sensory perception—were representative of ultimate Yang, or Heaven. On a perceptual (but not necessarily sensorial) level, these phenomena included the superconscious experience of deep meditation and the effects of celestial influences on the Earth. Based on their perception of the interrelatedness of all things, the Chinese developed a very sophisticated astrological science to elucidate the effects of the Heavens upon the Earth. In physical terms this science relates the effects of the sun and moon to the movement of earthly fluids, most apparent in the ceaselessly shifting rhythm of the tides. No less important, however, were the energetic effects of these heavenly influences on people's lives. Oriental bodywork treatment protocols involving the day of the week, the time of day, and even the selection of herbs or acupoints were all dependent upon astrological considerations unique to each individual.

The ancient sages considered the Earth itself to represent the great Yin pole of the cosmic Dao—our womb, our playground, the tapestry on and from which we weave the fabric of our daily lives, and ultimately our grave. All of the Ten Thousand Things are contained within the Sphere of Earth.[5]

The Spheres of Heaven and Earth are mutually dependent. They interpenetrate and interact with each other in a way that may be visualized in figure 2.2.[6]

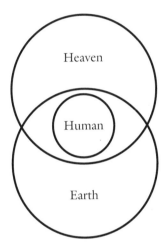

Fig. 2.2. Heaven ↔ Human ↔ Earth

The Chinese conceived the Sphere of the Human to be the realm of interaction between Heaven and Earth, with the Human (the person) influenced by and influencing both. The visceral processes by which we digest, assimilate, and eliminate food; our somatic makeup and vital energies; our personality development; our feelings; our internal and external, personal and political relationships—these are but some of the countless forms of Yin-Yang interaction that define human life.

On a more subtle level, the constant interpenetration and subsequent permutation of the Earth's geomagnetosphere by the electromagnetic fields of both the moon and the sun (the Sphere of Heaven)

cause a constant micropulsatory variation within the larger magnetic field of the Earth. The human organism, evolving within this constantly shifting field for mega-millennia, has adapted to this background clock as a means of timing its own internal biorhythmic changes, such as the wake-sleep cycle, temperature variations, menstruation, melatonin/serotonin production, and physical, mental, and emotional vitality.[7] Rapid alterations in the magnetic field wreak havoc with our internal rhythms, as any jet traveler can attest. Even the temporary and partial disengagement from the geomagnetic sphere caused by the magnetic interference of the countless steel cars, trains, ships, planes, and the high-rise buildings within which we spend so much time have been shown by Japanese researchers to create an imbalance in human biorhythmic systems.[8] Frequent alterations in our interaction with the Earth's geomagnetic field create the medically insoluble problems of low-level malaise and general aches and pains from which so many people suffer. In Japan there is a growing over-the-counter industry in magnetic ornaments and jewelry to remedy this problem.[9] Animal research in the United States has shown that extended insulation from the Earth's geomagnetic field produces confusion, lowered vitality, abnormal behavior, increased susceptibility to disease, increased mortality, and a progressive inability to successfully reproduce.[10] This situation represents a serious threat to our health, both individually and culturally.

SEASONS AND ELEMENTS

Within the constant dance of manifestation, Yin and Yang undergo five elementary transformations both in the world at large and in the human organism. The Five Element theory represents an approach to comprehending and managing the energetic balances created by this interaction of Heaven and Earth. The Five Element schemata represents a mnemonic device developed to correlate events taking place within the human ecology with the events taking place in the world.

Two keys will help us understand the Five Element theory. The first lies in recognizing the powerful naturalist tendencies of the Chinese scientist-philosophers. For them, the field of scientific observation was the phenomenal world, and the instruments of observation were the human mind and senses. They explored the nature of reality by observing the play of events in the world. Detailed observations made with still and collected minds, over long periods of time, uncovered certain patterns, or cycles, that allowed a wise person to live in accordance with nature. This focus on natural events predisposed them to a fluid and interactive, function-oriented perspective on the events they observed.

The second key lies in understanding the absolutely relative nature of the ancient Chinese perception of reality. For them there was no separation between self and world, or between mind and matter. Microcosm and macrocosm were totally related images of each other, reflecting and affecting each other in every particular.

Observation of the cycles of nature revealed a regular pattern to the changes of season. Based on their fivefold view of pattern evolution, the Chinese perceived five seasons—spring, summer, long summer, autumn, and winter. They noticed that, coincident with the seasons, all living things followed a cycle of birth, growth, maturity, withdrawal, and dormancy. They saw that the Earth renewed itself in the season of spring. Plants sprouted and then grew furiously. A fresh wind blew in from the east and cleared the air. The world turned blue-green and came to vibrant life. Then in the summer, the world turned hot. The sun

shone brightly from the south, and the peoples' skin turned red. The world grew lush and ripe.

At the end of summer, before the waning of autumn, the world became still. A humid pale settled on the land as the crops came to maturity and began to yellow. The land seemed to become the center of the universe.

In autumn the world dried out. The sun turned to the west. The rinds and skins of the crops began to whiten as an indication of their readiness for harvest. The world started to withdraw from the hectic pace of summer, preparing to hibernate. Then came winter, when the world turned cold and the sun shone weakly from the north. The sky became black. Life turned inward and became quiescent, silently beginning to germinate in preparation for the coming spring.

As the world, so too the people. Events in the macrocosm mirrored events in their personal lives. The same cycles that described and predicted the comings and goings of the world were seen to describe the inner workings of human life. Unlike the structurally differentiated elements of the Greco-Roman or Aryan cultures,[11] the Chinese derived a functional viewpoint of the elements that reflected the cycles of their world as it endlessly moved through its timeless changes.

The crossroads where the phases of life changed or transformed were called the Five Elements or Five Transformations: Fire, Earth, Metal, Water, and Wood. The Chinese sages developed this symbology describing the stages of transformation and used it as a mnemonic device to aid in remembering the countless signs, symptoms, and changes that corresponded—in the world, as in the individual human life—to each season. These signs of transformation include changes in mental, emotional, and physical symptomology, all related to the interplay of the Five Elements within the broader Yin-Yang dynamic.

Table 2.1 shows some of the basic divisions of general phenomena, body regions, tissues and organs, and other physiological activities in terms of the Five Elements.

The first known medical application of the Five Element theory occurs in the *Huang Di Nei Jing Su Wen,* believed to have been written at about the first century B.C.E. It was at this time that the descriptive framework of the eight trigrams,[12] used in the I Jing to describe the place of mankind in the world, began evolving into the Five Phase description of nature that has come down to us today. In the *Su Wen* the Yellow Emperor asks his chief physician, Qi Bo, "There are eight winds in Heaven and only five in the body, how is this?" Qi Bo answered, "The eight winds make evil; using the meridian Qi the eight winds can approach and touch the five Yin organs. Then the evil Qi makes disease."

Kiiko Matsumoto and Stephen Birch are two present-day acupuncturists at the forefront of the current effort to publish accurate English translations of traditional Oriental medical texts. In examining the transition from the trigrams to the Five Element theory, Matsumoto and Birch conjecture that the hexagrams dropped from the descriptive grid of the I Jing indicate the sages' perception of the essential imbalance inherent within the human condition. They point to the three dropped hexagrams as instructions for correcting this imbalance through the Daoist meditative practice of "Sitting still, slowly breathing"[13] (fig. 2.3).

The *Ling Shu* (Spiritual axis), a portion of the *Nei Jing* dated slightly later than the *Su Wen,* further developed the correlations between human life and the Five Element theory.[14] The last, and certainly the most detailed and complete, of the original source texts from which the Five Element theory has evolved is the *Nan Jing* (Classic of difficult questions). Its author undertook correlating and resolving, in eighty-one questions, the conflicting

TABLE 2.1

Basic Correspondences

SEASONAL CORRESPONDENCES					
	Wood	**Fire**	**Earth**	**Metal**	**Water**
Direction	East	South	Center	West	North
Seasons	Spring	Summer	Long summer	Autumn	Winter
Climactic Influence	Wind	Heat	Damp	Dryness	Cold

ORGAN CORRESPONDENCES					
	Wood	**Fire**	**Earth**	**Metal**	**Water**
Yin Organs	Liver	Heart	Spleen	Lung	Kidney
Yang Organs	Gallbladder	Small Intestine	Stomach	Large Intestine	Bladder
Effects	Blood	Consciousness	Flesh	Qi	Will
Yin Organs Store	Blood	Vessels	Nutritive Qi	Qi	Essence
Opens into	Eyes	Tongue	Lips	Nose	Ears or the 2 Yin
Branches into	Nails	Face color	Lips	Skin/Body hair	Head hair

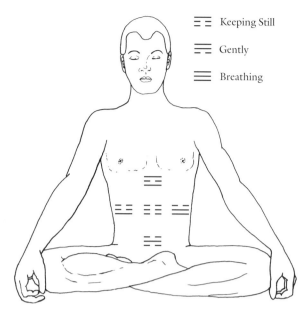

Keeping Still

Gently

Breathing

Fig. 2.3. The Three Trigrams Describing Meditation

theoretical information contained in the *Su Wen* and *Ling Shu*. Even so, we are left with certain paradoxes and difficulties of interpretation, reminding us that the Five Element theory provides a soft focus for problem solving when considering the human condition; it should not be mistaken for a rigid set of laws defining all energetic interactions. Rather, the theory points to probable tendencies, ones that may be profitably considered but that must be discarded in favor of other evaluation and treatment strategies if they fail to effectively address the issues under consideration.[15]

STEMS AND BRANCHES

As ultimate reality condenses from formlessness into form during the gestation of a human body, we can delineate a series of stages marking the descent from Heaven to Earth. Formlessness yields the Dao, which divides into Yin and Yang. These manifest as the Organ-Elements (see footnote on page 23), which further divide into Yin and Yang

Organs. The Yin components manifest as our internal viscera and their related pathways; the Yang components become our bowel organs and their pathways. This division of the Elements into their Yin-Yang polarities is called the Ten Celestial Stems. The Ten Stems represent an intermediate step between the Elements and their physical manifestation (fig. 2.4). The Branches are the last, and most concrete, stage of physical manifestation. They manifest as the twelve Organ-Element meridians that are addressed in our treatments.[16]

A major factor involved in maintaining balance between the cycles of transformation involves the Yin-Yang polarity of the internal Organs related to each Element. When a Yang Organ is overactive the complimentary Yin Organ becomes less active; when Yin function ascends, Yang activity depresses. This complementarity of Yin-Yang balance between related Organs is always operative.

The Chinese noticed that all of our internal Organs function in Element-related pairs: a visceral (Yin) Organ is always functionally coupled with a bowel (Yang) Organ. Thus, the Lung (Yin)

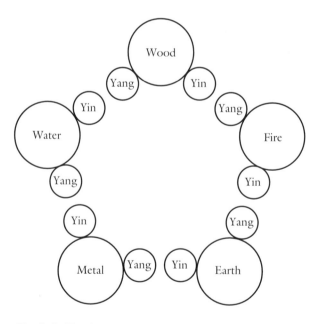

Fig. 2.4. Ten Stems

is functionally related to the Large Intestine (Yang). (We will discuss the Organs in greater detail in chapter 4.)

The Yang / Yin Organ pairings are as follows:

TABLE 2.2
Yang Organ / Yin Organ

Large Intestine (LI) / Lung (Lu)	LI/Lu
Stomach (St) / Spleen (Pancreas) (Sp)	St/Sp
Small Intestine (SI) / Heart (Ht)	SI/Ht
Bladder (Bl) / Kidney (Ki)	Bl/Ki
Gallbladder (Gb) / Liver (Li)	Gb/Li
Triple Heater (TH) / Heart Envelope (HE)	TH/HE

The list above shows that the spleen and pancreas are referred to as one Organ function, called the Spleen. The functional nature of the Chinese view of the internal Organs makes for no differentiation between the spleen and pancreas, which they considered as one gestalt responsible for the formation and control of blood, as well as the digestion of food and the movement of food Qi.

The Chinese identified two functions, in addition to the Organ systems paired with the organs of Western physiology, that may or may not correspond to actual physical structures but do clearly define and describe essential operations taking place within the body. These two functions also have their own meridians and acupoints. The Triple Heater is named for the distinct respiratory, digestive, and eliminative functions it controls. The Triple Heater also refers to the microtubular fluid circulatory system that carries intercellular fluids throughout our bodies, thus its traditional reference as "the sluices of the body."[17] The Triple Heater also serves to bring the root energy, or Source Qi, from the dan tien to the source points of the Organ meridians in two-hour intervals, helping to energize Organ functions.

The Chinese named the function that protects and supports the heart and controls our emotional and relational interactions the Heart Envelope. The Heart Envelope also refers to the whole mediastinal cavity, and by extension to the entire circulatory system.[18] This function is also called the heart constrictor, the pericardium, and the Circulation-Sex Meridian.

Properly speaking, the Triple Heater and Heart Envelope functions belong to an entirely different order of our energetic structure than the Organ/meridian system; they exist on a more basic energetic strata than the Five Element framework. Their functional rather than structural nature, and the different energetic qualities they manifest, have proven the source of much misunderstanding regarding their placement in the Five Element schematic. In daily life they pertain more to the energetic functions of the body than to the physical structure. In terms of the cycles of Creation and Control they are classified as accessory Fire Organs, and categorized as an aspect of the Fire Element.

CREATION AND CONTROL

There are two opposing but complementary tendencies responsible for maintaining balance within the Five Phase transformations. In the Creation Cycle:

- Wood *tends to* create Fire
- Fire *tends to* create Earth
- Earth *tends to* create Metal
- Metal *tends to* create Water
- Water *tends to* create Wood.

The balance for the Creation Cycle is the Control Cycle. In the Control Cycle:

- Wood *tends to* control Earth
- Earth *tends to* control Water
- Water *tends to* control Fire
- Fire *tends to* control Metal
- Metal *tends to* control Wood.

The Cycles of Creation and Control are represented in figure 2.5. The outer arrows trace the Creation Cycle; the arrows on the inside point from the controlling Element to that which it controls. Although these energetic tendencies represent the natural means by which the body maintains balance among its component parts, they also describe one of the probable pathways that imbalances follow as they ramify through the human system. The schema for the Creation and Control Cycles, along with the physical correspondences to the Five Elements, represent a powerful tool for medical diagnosis and prognosis, as well as for the design of wholistic treatment protocols.

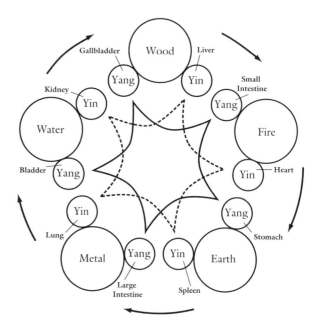

Fig. 2.6. *Organ Relationship in the Creation Cycle*

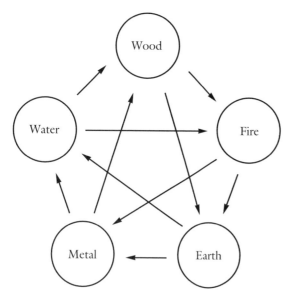

Fig. 2.5. *Cycles of Creation and Control*

In the Creation Cycle, each Yang Organ "creates" or nourishes the following Yang Organ, and each Yin Organ nourishes the following Yin Organ

(fig. 2.6). Left to itself, the Creation Cycle would cause the system to move toward ever greater excess, with the Elements creating each other in an endlessly increasing circle. This obviously is not what happens. The increase in each quality is checked by the Control Cycle, in which each Yin Organ balances the Yin Organ of the Element it controls; likewise, each Yang Organ balances the Yang Organ of the Element it controls (fig. 2.7). Also significant is the balancing effect of Element-related Yin and Yang Organs upon each other. The balancing effect between the Yin and Yang Organs of each Element in the control cycle works in both directions. Imbalance in either partner can affect the other.

OVERWHELM AND REBELLION

The Cycles of Creation and Control describe the tendencies of the human system when it is operating in a balanced fashion. Pathological manifesta-

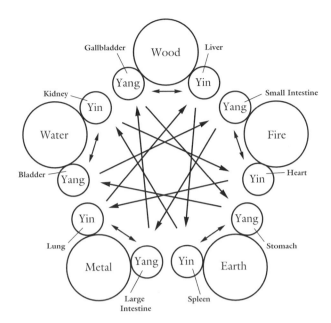

Fig. 2.7. Organ Relationship in the Control Cycle

tions occur when these mechanisms are not functioning optimally. When one of the Organ phases becomes depleted, the normal Organ-phase function controlling it can further weaken and overwhelm it. For example, Water normally regulates Fire, but if the Fire isn't hot enough, even slight moistening can put it out. In organic terms, the Kidney controls the Heart, but if the Heart's function is already inadequate, normal Kidney control can overwhelm it. The only difference between the Cycle of Control and the Cycle of Overwhelm is one of proportion. Normal action, in the presence of prior weakness, can produce disproportionate influence.

A second possibility for inappropriate interaction between Organ-Elements occurs when one phase or Organ is so excessive that it rebels against the Organ phase that normally controls it, harming that controlling Organ. For example, an extremely overactive Liver can "scorch" and weaken the functioning of the Lung, which normally keeps Liver function under control.

From an energetic viewpoint, *disease* can be described as any impediment to the free flow of vital energy. What determines whether or not a shift in energetic balance will precipitate disease is the preexisting harmony of the system before it is stressed. The human organism is blessed with amazing recuperative power; the body most frequently absorbs and redistributes offensive stimuli, going about the normal process of continual transformation with no symptoms whatsoever. It is only in circumstances of preexisting disharmony that further energetic imbalance can result in disease.

Whether or not there is pain, dysfunction, or degeneration, the disease process is an indication of the excesses and/or deficiencies in our various bodily systems. It is not energetic transformation per se, but unpleasant transformation—changes that include consequences we do not like—that we call disease. The Five Element paradigm gives us a highly probable, though not infallible, guide to both the tendencies of transformation and the method of recreating balance in the bodymind.

CORRESPONDENCES

Chinese medical science, as discussed earlier, is basically preventive in nature. Although the ancient Chinese physician/scientists developed an extensive repertoire of treatments for specific diseases, the Great Healer treated disease states before they manifested. The remediation of actual pathology was the province of the mediocre physician. This rather remarkable goal was accomplished by assiduous observation. All of the signs and symptoms that accompanied each stage of the process of imbalance leading to disease and the corresponding events that occurred with them were noted by the Chinese physicians. This system enabled them to recognize all of the many patterns that manifest in the evolution of disease. They were able to tailor their treatments individually from the very onset of the degenerative process based on this system of predictive pattern recognition, rather than waiting for actual pathology to herald the need for treatment.

Western medicine requires a specific diagnosis and name for each "disease" before treatment begins. Eastern medicine, on the other hand, recognizes that many different kinds of underlying imbalance can result in similar sets of symptoms. Effective remediation of root causes can only follow from an accurate assessment of the total energetic picture. The presenting symptoms of the patient become secondary in this process, as layers of root imbalance can be totally asymptomatic. A total energetic assessment—through truly skillful use of the presenting signs and symptoms as well as their known correspondences—is what allows the Great Healer to identify and correct imbalances before they manifest as disease.

All of the information, conscious and unconscious, that a client brings to a practitioner must be integrated into a cohesive pattern. Effective treatment aimed at the recreation of true energetic balance requires a more profound and subtle understanding of the total "landscape" than is required for merely remediating symptoms. The first step, however, must be to address each client's presenting complaints. Great pain, for example, requires immediate treatment; the background patterns of the entire system cannot even begin to be discerned until it is treated.

The main categories used for the Element correspondences include the Organ/meridians; their character; the time they are most active; the season of the year that affects them the most; climatological effects; emotional correspondences; related color changes; relevant odors; taste preferences in food that aid or harm the Organs; the way speech patterns are affected; related sense organs, bodily fluids, areas of the body, and physiological functions of the organs themselves; the effects on the Essential Substances; changes in the tongue and radial pulses; and the effects on individual consciousness. There are several excellent books that discuss these correspondences in great detail.[19]

CHAPTER 3

ORIENTAL PHYSIOLOGY: THE ESSENTIAL SUBSTANCES AND INTERNAL ORGANS

THE ESSENTIAL SUBSTANCES may be considered the heart of Oriental physiology. Produced by the Yin and Yang Organs, these Substances are fundamental to maintaining a person's health and vigor. Five in number, the Essential Substances are:

- Qi
- Xue (Blood)
- Jing (Essence)
- Shen (Consciousness)
- Jin-ye (Fluids)

Jing, Qi, and Shen form a continuum. They are the essential manifestations of the Heaven↔Human↔Earth triad (fig. 3.1). Jing (Essence) is the most Yin of the Essential Substances. A liquid residing in the Kidney,* in the Lower Heater, Jing forms the basis of the physical manifestation of the body. Qi, which is Yang in nature and fuels all activ-

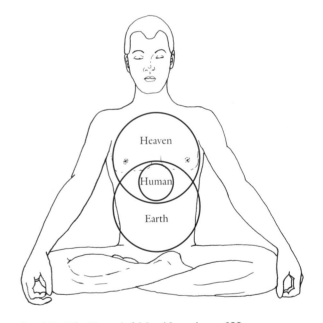

Fig. 3.1. The Essential Manifestations of Heaven ↔ Human ↔ Earth

ity of the body, ultimately derives from Jing and is a more rarefied Substance. It has its source in the

---

*In this text I will be following the Oriental medical tradition of referring to each Organ in the singular. When the subject under discussion is a broad concept of Oriental medicine, the words will appear with an initial capital; this includes all references to an Organ as a functional/energetic unit. When the subject under discussion is the material organ body, the word will appear in all lower-case letters.

Middle Heater in the Spleen and Stomach. Not material in Western terms, Shen (Consciousness) is the most rarefied Substance of all. Rooted in the Jing and Qi, it resides in the Upper Heater in the Heart. This triad, referred to as the Three Treasures, is considered the essence of human nature.

The Substances are also distinguished as sets of complementary polarities. Qi and Blood are seen as inseparable aspects of a Yin-Yang gradient, as are Essence and Consciousness. Traditionally the Fluids were also separated into a polar pair and discussed as Yang Liquids and Yin Humors. As in all things, the Chinese distinguished the Yin-Yang complementarity of each pair, differentiating the quantitative Yin structure from the qualitative Yang function.

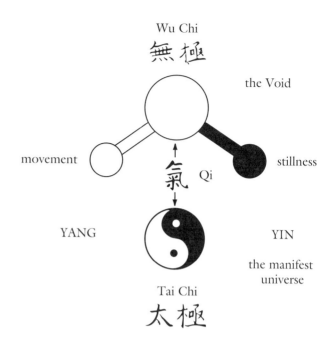

Fig. 3.2. Wu Chi–Tai Chi–Qi Continuum

Q I

In the science of traditional Chinese medicine (TCM), Qi is considered the fundamental particle/wave of the manifest universe. In Chinese cosmology, after Yin and Yang separate from the unmanifest void of Wu Chi, which is the equivalent of the Christian concept of God Transcendent, and begin to interact as Tai Chi, the equivalent of God imminent, the first manifestation is Qi (fig. 3.2). The *Huai Nan Zi* (Book of Master Huai Nan) (c. 122 B.C.E.) says:

> Dao originated from Emptiness and Emptiness produced the universe. The Universe produced Qi. . . . That which was clear and light drifted up to become Heaven, and that which was heavy and turbid solidified to become Earth.[1]

Yang in nature, Qi represents the basic motive power of the universe. It has been variously translated as energy, material force, ether, matter-

energy, vital force, life force, vital power, and moving power. The literal translation of the ideogram shows the character for uncooked rice covered by the character for steam or gas (fig. 3.3). This indicates both the dual, material-immaterial nature of Qi as well as its root in the digestive processes of the body.

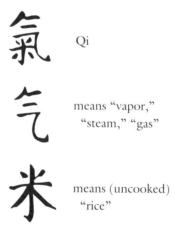

Qi

means "vapor," "steam," "gas"

means (uncooked) "rice"

Fig. 3.3. Qi

Essentially, Qi is the Chinese equivalent of our modern concept of the matter-energy continuum or the electromagnetic spectrum. Very early in their study of the nature of reality, the Chinese recognized that matter and energy were merely different states of the same fundamental basic substance. Zhang Zai (1020–1077 C.E.) said:

> The Great Void consists of Qi. Qi condenses to become the ten thousand things. Things of necessity disintegrate and return to the Great Void. . . . Qi in dispersion is substance, and so is it in condensation. . . . Every birth is a condensation, every death is a dispersal. Birth is not a gain, death not a loss. . . . When condensed, Qi becomes a living being. When dispersed, it is the substratum of mutations.[2]

Because they regarded all phenomena, from the most dense "matter" to the most rarefied consciousness, as different states of condensation of Qi, in constant mutation from one form to another and from form to formlessness and back again, their science never foundered on the Cartesian rock of separating energy or life from matter. All manifestation was seen as Qi in varying states of condensation or dispersal. When dispersed it forms the Great Void, the subatomic matrix of the universe. When condensed it forms all phenomena of the universe, from consciousness to the most inert matter.

The human form is a manifestation of condensed Qi. The economy of the human energetic system is funded by two interrelated sources. Prenatal or Ancestral Qi, also called the Qi of Heaven or Jing, is inherited from our parents. Prenatal Qi may be likened to a trust fund: we may not draw from it directly, but it constantly works to help maintain our daily bank balance. Prenatal Qi determines our genetic makeup and general state of health, although the Chinese concept of Prenatal

Qi is not identical to the Western concept of genetic inheritance. Genetic consequences are generally limited to the physical reproduction of bodies in a time-bound sequence, while the transmission of Prenatal Qi may well involve karmic factors[3] not accounted for by the genomes transmitted from parent to child.

The second energy source for human life is called Postnatal or Acquired Qi, or the Qi of Earth. Derived from water, food, and air, this Qi represents the pocket money that we use for our daily expenses. The *Su Wen* says, "A human being results from the Qi of Heaven and Earth. . . . The union of the Qi of Heaven and Earth is called human being."[4] The *Nan Jing* says, "Qi is the root of a human being."[5] Qi is the fundamental Substance from which all other aspects of the human being derive.

Qi may be said to have five basic functions:

1. Activating: Qi activates all of our bodily processes, fueling growth, development, and metabolism.
2. Warming: Qi maintains body temperature.
3. Defending: Qi controls the immune function.
4. Transforming: Qi mediates the production of Blood, Humors, and Fluids, their distribution throughout the body, and their conversion into urine and sweat.
5. Containing: Qi contains our internal Fluids as needed, preventing extravasation of the Blood or excessive perspiration or urination. This function of Qi also keeps the internal organs in their proper places, preventing them from prolapsing.

In order to facilitate discussion, Western physiology uses different names to characterize the various aspects of the single basic fluid that flows within our bodies, both inside and outside the blood vessels and lymph channels. The Chinese took the same approach in describing the various functions of Qi within the body.

In Chinese medicine Qi has two major aspects. First, it refers to the refined essence, produced by each of the Organs, that nourishes the body and mind. This basic form of Qi is called by various names according to its location or activity, as in Source Qi or Food Qi. Secondly, Qi refers to the functional activity of the Organs. Thus Lung Qi points to the activities of the Lung—circulating Defensive Qi under the skin—not to a substance stored or produced in the Lung. Each distinct manifestation of the different physiological processes of Qi is recognized as a function of Original Qi and given its own name.

Pre-Heaven Qi (Yuan Qi)

Yuan Qi is the original distillation of the liquid Jing (Essence) as it sublimes into Qi. This transformation takes place in the Kidney, or rather in the space between the kidneys, which is also called the Gate of Vitality or Ming Men. Yuan Qi both feeds and is fed by the Post-Heaven Qi of digestion. The Yuan Qi includes Original Yin and Original Yang, as it is the foundation of all of the energies in the body.

Yuan Qi fundamentally arouses and activates the various functions of the internal Organs. As the essence of Qi itself, it motivates every activity. It is the basis for Kidney Qi, and thus provides the heat necessary for every transformation in the body. Yuan Qi is essential for the conversion of Food Qi and Air Qi into True Qi in the Lung or Blood in the Heart. Yuan Qi is the Qi that the Triple Heater Meridian brings from the Source to each channel in the Creation Cycle, and that comes out at the Source points and energizes the activities of each Organ at a specific time of day.

Post-Heaven Qi

FOOD QI (GU QI)

Food and water enter the Stomach in the Middle Heater, where they are rotted and ripened and then converted into Gu Qi by the transforming power of the Spleen.

CHEST QI (ZONG QI)

Not yet in a form usable by the body, Food Qi is transported by the Spleen to the Upper Heater where it is combined with the Breath (Da) Qi of the Lung to form Ancestral Qi (Zong Qi), also known as Gathering Qi,[6] Chest Qi, or Big Qi. Zong Qi resides in the chest, powering respiration, and is essential in the further transformation of Food Qi into True Qi or Blood. The *Su Wen* characterizes the Zong Qi as ". . . the energy that comes out under the left breast and can be felt under the fingers."[7] Zong Qi has several functions having to do with nourishing the Heart and Lung. It is responsible for driving both the pulse and respiration, giving strength to both as well as to the voice. It is also responsible for transporting Qi to the lower portion of the body, thus connecting the Lung and Kidney. The area of the chest where Zong Qi gathers is called the sea of Qi, and is controlled by the Conception Vessel (CV) 17 acupoint.

TRUE QI (ZHEN QI).

When Yuan Qi is added to Zong Qi, Zhen or True Qi results. This is the final form of Qi that flows in the channels. True Qi assumes two different forms according to its Yin or Yang nature; these forms are called Ying or Nutritive Qi, and Wei or Defensive Qi. Nutritive Qi is the finer essence of True Qi. Yin in nature, Ying Qi flows with the Blood and provides nourishment to the entire body. Defensive Qi is the coarser part of the True Qi. More Yang than the Nutritive Qi, it circulates between the skin and muscles and serves to protect us from external pathogens. Wei Qi represents the superficial functions of our immune system (i.e., the functions we assign to the various white blood cells that protect us from infection when the skin is broken); it also serves to open and close the pores and keep the skin moist and supple. The *Su Wen* tells us that "Defensive Qi is the fierce Qi of the digestate."[8]

Other names for different aspects or functions of Qi are:

CENTRAL QI (ZHONG QI)
Central Qi is the root of Post-Heaven Qi in the Middle Heater.

CORRECT QI (ZHENG QI)
Correct Qi refers to the appropriate function of the Wei Qi in defending the exterior from pathogenic invasion.

ORGAN QI (ZANG-FU QI)
Organ Qi represents the motive force behind the physiological functions performed by the viscera and bowels.

CHANNEL QI (JING-LUO QI)
Channel Qi flows through the pathways, enabling communication between the internal organs and energizing the surface of the body. The sensation produced when stimulating an acupoint, called "obtaining the Qi," is a manifestation of Channel Qi. This is the Qi that is activated through finger pressure in a shiatsu/anma treatment.

XUE (BLOOD)

In TCM, Blood is a much different substance than its Western counterpart. Blood is a form of Qi, the most dense and Yin aspect of Qi in the body, but part of a spectrum that runs from the most rarefied Qi, Shen, to Blood. All of the Essential Substances are ultimately made of Qi.

Blood is formed from the Food Qi of the Stomach and Spleen, which the Lung pushes to the Heart. Here it is combined with the Source Qi derived from the Kidney Essence and so transformed into Blood by the Fire of the Heart. Qi and Blood are inseparable, as Ying (Nutritive) Qi flows with the blood through every vessel, performing the Yin function of nourishing and moistening all the tissues of the body. Blood also houses the Qi and the Shen, providing the material substrate necessary for both Qi and Shen to have a root in the body. The red, physical liquid we call blood is only a portion of the physical-energetic spectrum the Chinese call Blood.

The various forms of Qi within the body are responsible for the three functions of production, circulation, and containment of the Blood, and for this reason Qi is known as the commander of the Blood. Blood, though, is known as the mother of Qi, as it is only through proper nourishment being brought to all parts of the body that Qi is generated. Describing these interdependent qualities that form the basis of active life, the *Nan Jing* states: "Qi invigorates, and Blood nourishes."[9] And according to the *Su Wen:* "If Qi and Blood fall into disharmony, a hundred diseases may arise."[10]

After Blood is formed by the heat of Heart Fire infusing the Food Qi from the Spleen with Source Qi, the Heart pumps it throughout the body in concert with the Lung, which provides the Qi necessary for the proper function of the circulatory vessels.

JING AND SHEN (ESSENCE AND CONSCIOUSNESS)

The Chinese delineated Jing and Shen as two complementary poles of the energy that is primarily responsible for determining human growth and development, and for fueling activity and metabolism. These two polar complements describe the Yin-Yang gradient within the human energetic experience. According to the ancient texts, the Heart is the abode of Shen; the Kidney is the storehouse of Jing.[11] Jing is the earthy, Yin aspect of our energy, derived from food and water. Shen is the more rarefied Yang Qi derived from the breath. The *Huai Nan Zi* states that "Jing is the Qi of the person" and "Shen is the protective nature of the person."[12] Jing refers to the energy involved in the process of creating the actual physical form and to the vitality energizing it. Shen refers to the more subtle activity of mind or spirit. Shen is intimately involved with our emotions. Balanced and abundant Shen fills the heart and causes all of the seven emotions to remain in balance.

Our ability to reproduce is a direct function of Jing. If the acquired Essence of the Organs is abundant, then the Kidney can store the surplus and convert it into reproductive essence, which becomes the congenital Essence that is passed on to our offspring. This TCM understanding of original Essence has profound implications with regard to our notions about genetic inheritance.

Blood and Essence form a reciprocal relationship of mutual nourishment, and they can convert into one another when necessary. Kidney Essence produces Marrow, which in turn generates the bone marrow that contributes to the formation of Blood, especially in the resting state when the Blood has been returned to the Liver to be replenished and stored. For this reason it is said that Liver and Kidney have the same source, and that Blood is transformed from Kidney Essence.

JIN-YE FLUIDS (LIQUIDS AND HUMORS)

This category of the Essential Substances refers to all the fluids within the body other than Blood and Jing. Again, considered as a continuum, Liquids are the Yang aspect, being relatively thin and mobile. Humors, the thicker, more viscous secretions of the organs, are recognized as the Yin aspect of Fluids. The Liquids are mostly found on the surface of the body, moisturizing flesh, skin, hair, and the mucous membranes of the special senses. Liquids also perform a cleansing action, allowing the body to detoxify through the elimination of fluids, via sweat and urine. Humors are the fluids of organic processes and the lubricants of the joints.

THE FUNCTIONS OF THE INTERNAL ORGANS

The Chinese categorize the internal organs as Yin viscera (Zang) or Yang bowels (Fu). The Zang are defined as "organs that store," in reference to the role of the Yin Organs in storing the Essential Substances of Qi, Blood, Fluids, Essence, and Consciousness. Fu translates as "organs that act as the seat of government," referring to the Yang Organ function of transforming food and drink into Blood and Qi. The Zang are solid organs of constant function and are essential for life. The Fu are hollow organs of intermittent function; life can continue in their absence. The *Su Wen* says:

> The five Yin Organs store Essence and Qi and do not excrete: they can be full but not

in Excess. The six Yang Organs transform and digest and do not store: they can be in Excess but not full. In fact, after food enters the mouth, the Stomach is full and the Intestines are empty; when the food goes down, the Intestines are full and the Stomach is empty.[13]

The Yin Organs store the refined Essential Substances, necessary for the maintenance of vitality, which the Yang Organs transform from food, drink, and air. Each Substance is related to particular Organs. The Heart governs the Blood and the Liver stores the Blood. The Lung governs Qi and influences Fluids. The Spleen governs Food Qi, holds the Blood in the channels, and transforms and transports Fluids. The Kidney stores Essence and excretes Fluids.

The Yang Organs, on the other hand, are constantly being filled and emptied as they extract and refine the Essential Substances that the Yin Organs store. Yang Organ functions serve to receive, move, transform, and digest food and excrete waste. Each Yang Organ is likened to a particular government office, reflecting the importance of its particular role in the production of the Essential Substances for which it is responsible.

The Yin viscera and Yang bowels are paired according to their elementary natures. The internal/external relationship between viscus and bowel is considered to be structural as well as functional. The Yin Organs are the structural component of each organ/bowel dyad, storing the Vital Substances, while the Yang Organs may be considered as the functional aspect, moving, producing, and excreting these substances. Each internal viscera is connected via the meridian system to its related external bowel, with the flow of Qi energizing them sequentially throughout the day. The functions of these dyads are related to each other, some more closely than others. For example, it is easy to recognize the relationships between the Kidney and the Bladder, the Stomach and Spleen (Pancreas), or the Liver and Gallbladder. The relationship between the Lung and Large Intestine is not so obvious—both play an eliminative role in the body. An even more subtle pairing is that between the Heart and the Small Intestine—their functional relationship pertains to the twin fires of circulation and digestion.

While Western medicine focuses on the physical structure of the organs, Chinese medicine focuses on the pattern of functions of the Organs. Although morphologically related to the organs recognized by Western medicine, functionally the sphere of affect of each of the Zang Fu is radically different from those of the Western organs. In fact, a Western practitioner would consider certain functions as being related to entirely different organs or systems than the Chinese. For example, emotional balance and clarity of mind, which Western medicine ascribes to the proper functioning of the nervous and endocrine systems, are considered to be controlled by the Heart and Heart Envelope Organ functions.

Because of their vital role in storing the Essential Substances, the Zang are considered primary in Chinese physiology. Each Zang Organ is in functional relationship with different tissues in the body. Thus the Heart controls the blood vessels and manifests in the complexion; the Liver controls the sinews and manifests in the nails; the Lung controls the skin and manifests in the body hair; the Spleen controls the muscles and manifests in the lips; the Kidney controls the bones and manifests in the hair on the head.

Every sense organ also relates to one of the Zang Organs, the health of the sense organ depending on the proper function of the Zang Organ. The Heart controls the tongue and speech; the Liver controls the eyes and sight; the Lung controls the nose and smell; the Spleen controls the mouth and taste; and the Kidney controls the ears and hearing. There is also a reciprocal relationship between the Organs and emotions, the state of the Organ affecting the emotions and the emotions affecting the health of that Organ. The Heart relates to joy, the Liver to anger, the Lung to sadness, the Spleen to excessive thought, and the Kidney to fear. Further, each Organ is particularly vulnerable to one of the climatalogical factors: heat influences the Heart; wind influences the Liver; dryness influences the Lung; dampness influences the Spleen; and cold influences the Kidney.

Finally, different aspects of consciousness are controlled by different Organs, in contradistinction to our Western considerations about the primacy of the brain in this arena. Thus the Heart is recognized as the seat of Consciousness (Shen), the Ethereal Soul (Hun) resides in the Liver, the Corporeal Soul (Po) is housed in the Lung, the Will (Zhi) is directed by the Kidney, and Thought (Yi) is controlled by the Spleen.

The relationships between the Zang Organs and the tissues, senses, emotions, and environment are used therapeutically for diagnosis, prognosis, and the creation of treatment protocol.

The Yin Organs

THE HEART (XIN)

The *Ling Shu* says, "The Heart is the monarch of the five Yin Organs and the six Yang Organs and it is the residence of Shen."[14] Because it is the residence of Shen (consciousness) and because of its governance of Blood, the Heart is named the monarch of the Organs. It is said to govern the Blood because it is in the Heart that the Qi of digestion and respiration are combined with the Original Qi of the Kidney to form Blood. The Heart is primarily responsible for circulation and also controls the health of the blood vessels. As the home of consciousness, a healthy Heart is prerequisite for the proper function of the mental and emotional functions of joy and a balanced emotional life, as well as awareness, memory, thought, and sleep. The Heart opens into the tongue and controls speech, hence its condition is readily apparent in the appearance of the tongue. The Heart also controls perspiration.

THE LIVER (GAN)

The *Su Wen* states, "The Liver is like an army's general from whom strategy is derived."[15] The Liver accomplishes this responsibility for strategic planning by insuring smoothness and proper direction to the flow of Qi throughout the body. Since imbalance in both the Organs and the emotions begins with the restricted or misdirected flow of Qi, this function is critical to good health. Proper digestion is also dependent on the free and appropriate flow of Qi. The Liver stores and cleans the Blood when we lie down, returning it to the muscles when we are active. Adequate Blood storage also regulates and controls normal menstruation. The Liver controls the sinews as the strength and pliability of both ligaments and tendons are dependent on adequate moisture and nourishment from the Liver Blood. The Liver manifests in the nails, which become dry and brittle when Liver Blood is out of balance. The Liver opens into the eyes, which immediately reflect the health of the Liver. Finally, the Liver houses the Hun (Ethereal Soul), the equivalent of the Christian concept of soul as the spiritual essence that survives the death of the body. Thus the Liver is the origin of courage, resoluteness, clarity of purpose, direction, and creative drive.

THE LUNG (FEI)

The *Su Wen* calls the Lung "a minister from whom policies are issued."[16] This entitlement comes from the part it plays in aiding the Heart to control circulation. Although the Heart controls the condition of the blood vessels themselves, the circulation of Blood is driven by the Qi acquired by the Lung. The primary function of the Lung is governing Qi and respiration. It is the addition of Lung Qi to the Nutritive Qi of digestion that leads to the formation of True Qi in the Heart. Because Lung Qi is so essential for circulation in both the meridians and blood vessels we can determine the state of all of the internal Organs at the Lung Source point (Lu9) overlying the radial pulse of the wrist. The Lung also controls dispersing and descending. It is responsible for dispersing the Defensive (Wei) Qi from the Stomach evenly under the skin all over the body, thus protecting us from invasion by external pathogens. The Lung also disperses the bodily fluids that keep the skin moist and supple and control the opening and closing of the pores, and hence is said to control the skin and body hair. Because it is the uppermost Organ, the Lung is responsible for the descending function of both Qi and Fluids, connecting to the Kidney in the Lower Heater. As the Lung controls the orderly descent of Fluids from the Stomach to the Kidney and Bladder, it is said to control the water passages. The Lung opens into the nose and houses the Corporeal Soul (Po). The Chinese consider the Soul to have a Yang, spiritual aspect known as the Hun, which survives after the death of the body, and a Yin, physical aspect called the Po, which returns to the earth when the body dies. The Po corresponds to our concept of somatic intelligence, controlling movement and sensation.

THE SPLEEN (PI)

Of the Spleen the *Ling Shu* says: "The Spleen is the granary official from whom the five tastes are derived."[17] Its principle function, working in conjunction with the Stomach, is to transform and transport Food Qi in the process of making Qi and Blood. The Spleen controls the upward transportation of Food Qi to the Lung, where it combines with Breath Qi to form the Big Qi of the chest, and to the Heart, where it combines with Original Qi from the Kidney to form Blood. Thus, the Spleen is responsible for controlling the upward movement of Qi and for the transformation of Fluids. It is this control of the raising of Qi that prevents the internal organs from prolapsing. The Spleen also controls the muscles, especially in the limbs, by its control of the transport of Nutritive Qi throughout the body. Additionally, the Spleen controls the Blood, keeping it within its vessels as well as contributing to its formation. The Spleen opens into the mouth and lips and houses the Yi (thought), especially as thought relates to studying, concentrating, and memorizing. **Note:** The Chinese did not differentiate the pancreas as a separate organ, ascribing both its endocrine function of producing enzymes for the digestive process, as well as the exocrine function of insulin in bringing glycogen into the muscles, to the Spleen.

THE KIDNEY (SHEN)

The *Su Wen* says "The Kidney is the strong official from whom ingenuity is derived."[18] The Kidney forms the foundation of all of the other Organs. It is the repository of the Pre-Heaven Jing, which drives conception and fetal development, and after birth provides the Primary Yin and Primary Yang from which all Water and Fire in the body are derived. Kidney Yin is the fundamental substance upon which birth, growth, maturation, and reproduction depend, while Kidney Yang provides the energetic heat that fuels all of the physiological processes of the body. The primary function of the Kidney is to store Essence (Jing) and to govern birth, growth, maturation, and reproduction. Male Jing produces sperm, and female Jing produces the ovum. These combine to provide the

Pre-Heaven Essence of the child. Constitutional strength, vigor, sexual vitality, and the various stages of development are controlled by this Essence. Post-Heaven Essence, derived from the excess Essence produced by the other Organs from water, food, and air, is also stored in the Kidney and is responsible for sexual potency. The Kidney also produces Marrow, fills up the brain, and controls the bones. Marrow, a purely Chinese concept, is a potent precursor material, which in turn produces bone marrow and the central nervous system. For this reason the spinal cord and brain are called "the sea of Marrow," and are physiologically linked to the Kidney. This is the root of its appellation as the "official from whom ingenuity is derived." In addition to bones, Marrow also produces the teeth.

The Kidney governs Water, representing the Water element in the Five Element schema. Although the Lung, Spleen, Intestines, Bladder, and Triple Heater cooperate in regulating water in the body, all of these functions are driven by the heat of Kidney Yang. The Kidney also controls urination, opening and closing the "gate" of the Bladder. Thus the Kidney is said to control the two lower orifices, the urethra (including the spermatic duct in men), and the anus. Although anatomically related to the Large Intestine, the opening and closing of the anus is controlled by Kidney Yang. The Kidney controls the reception of Qi, holding Qi down after it is received by the Lung so that it may be utilized by the body. The Kidney opens into the ears and controls the hair on the head. The Kidney houses the Will (Zhi) and is responsible for our ability to remain focused on a goal until it is complete.

The Kidney is also the origin of Fire in the body. Organ theory (in contradistinction to Five Element theory) places the root of Fire in Ming Men, sometimes said to be the right kidney and sometimes said to lie between the kidneys. This is reflected in the placement of the Kidney at the left rear position of the radial pulse, while the energetic functions of the Heart Envelope and Triple Heater occupy the right rear position. (See pages 65–68 for more on the pulses.) Ming Men, the Gate of Vitality, is the root of the Source (Yuan) Qi, the first transformation of Essence into Qi, which is the source of Heat, the motive force for all physiological activity in the body. In addition, Yuan Qi, brought to the Source points of the meridians by the Triple Heater, helps the Nutritive Qi and Blood to move through the channels. While it may appear paradoxical to the Western mind to name the Kidney as the root of both Fire and Water, the Organ theory and Five Element theory, from which these concepts derive, have proved their validity over millennia of clinical practice.

THE HEART ENVELOPE (XIN BAO)

The Heart Envelope is not truly a separate Organ but rather the protective covering of the Heart, the pericardium. This is functionally extended to include the entire mediastinal cavity. The *Su Wen* consistently refers to the Five Yin and Six Yang Organs. In reference to the Heart Envelope it says, "If a pathogenic factor does attack the Heart, it will be diverted to attack the Heart Envelope instead."[19] While the Organ lacks a distinct medical function, the superficial meridian is the focus of treatment in acupuncture and bodywork for a host of somato-emotional conditions.

The Yang Organs

THE STOMACH (WEI)

The Stomach is unique in many ways, and is the most important of the Yang Organs. It is the only Yang Organ to play an equal role with its paired Yin Organ. The *Su Wen* says, "The Stomach and Spleen are the officials in charge of food storage and from whom the five flavors are derived."[20] The Stomach and Spleen are anomalous in Organ theory in that each performs tasks we would normally expect of an Organ of opposite polarity. The Stomach, a Yang Organ, is the origin of Fluids. Its Qi descends, it likes wetness, its channel is on the front of the body, and it frequently suffers from Yin Deficiency, all of which are Yin characteristics. The Spleen on the other hand, a Yin Organ, has the Yang function of transforming and transporting. Its Qi ascends, it likes dryness, and it can only suffer Deficient Yang. These characteristics are all Yang in nature. The Stomach and Spleen are so closely linked in their functions that they can be considered as the Yin-Yang polarity of a single digestive organ.

Food and water are transformed in the Stomach by a fermentation process the Chinese call "rotting and ripening." This is similar to the Western physiological description of the stomach as the site where ingested food is prepared for further digestion and assimilation. More importantly, the Stomach controls the transportation of food essences. While the Spleen directs the refined food essence to the various Organs, this function is entirely dependent on the motive power of Stomach Qi. The pulse is also powered by Stomach Qi. The thin, white coating normally seen on the surface of the tongue is indicative of adequate Stomach Qi. Stomach Qi is responsible for sending transformed food and fluids downward for further processing. When this is deficient, food and fluids stagnate in the Stomach. The Stomach is the origin of Fluids, as the Jin Ye originate here through the combined actions of the Kidney and Spleen. Excessive Stomach conditions can also profoundly affect the Shen, causing various kinds of manic behavior.

THE SMALL INTESTINE (XIAO CHANG)

Of the Small Intestine the *Su Wen* says, "The Small Intestine is the official in charge of receiving, being filled, and transforming."[21] It controls receiving and transforming as well as separating fluids. Thus, after the refined food essence in the Stomach is separated and extracted by the Spleen, the remaining digestate is passed on to the Small Intestine, which further separates the "clean" part from the "dirty" part. The clean part is then transported by the Spleen to nourish all of the tissues of the body, while the dirty part is transmitted to the Large Intestine or Bladder for elimination. The Small Intestine is responsible for mental clarity and sound judgment.

THE LARGE INTESTINE (DA CHANG)

The function of the Large Intestine is to receive the spent digestate from the Small Intestine, extract any remaining useful fluid, and eliminate the remains as stool. Traditional Chinese medical theory holds that the transporting function of the digestate through the Small and Large Intestines is controlled by the Spleen. The Large Intestine is paired with the Lung in Five Element theory, primarily because it is the descending function of Lung Qi that energizes defecation. Further, both Lung and Large Intestine are eliminative Organs.

THE GALLBLADDER (DAN)

The *Su Wen* calls the Gallbladder "The upright official that takes decisions."[22] The Gallbladder is unique among the Yang Organs in that it does not deal with food, drink, or waste products, or communicate with the exterior. Like a Yin Organ it functions to store a refined substance, bile, which it excretes to aid the Stomach and Spleen in digestion. This is identical to the Western medical viewpoint. The Gallbladder is called "the Yang of the Liver," helping to ensure the smooth flow of digestate just as the Liver ensures the smooth flow of Qi. As well, the Gallbladder cooperates with the Liver in controlling the sinews, providing them with Qi while the Liver nourishes them with Blood. The

Gallbladder also controls judgment, working together with the Liver to execute planning and activity. While the Liver controls our ability to make plans, the Gallbladder controls the courage and initiative to make decisions. In fact, the Chinese say an audacious person has "big gallbladder."

THE BLADDER (PANG GUANG)

The *Su Wen* says, "The Bladder is like a district official. It stores the Fluids so that they can be excreted by its action of Qi transformation."[23] The Bladder is considered to be the physical manifestation of Kidney Yang; it is from Ming Men that the Bladder derives the Qi and Heat needed to transform the dirty Fluids passed on by the Small Intestine into urine. Emotionally, Bladder dysfunction can manifest as jealousy, suspicion, and the tendency to hold a grudge.

THE TRIPLE HEATER (SAN JIAO)

The exact nature of the Triple Heater in Oriental physiology has been clouded in confusion for millennia. Although it is considered to be one of the Yang Organs, its exact functions, and even the question of whether it is an Organ at all, has fueled debate since the time of the *Nei Jing*. There are basically three different views of the Triple Heater, all of which we will consider here. The oldest viewpoint, elucidated in the *Su Wen*, is that the Triple Heater is one of the Yang Organs, with form as well as function. The *Su Wen* calls the Triple Heater "the official in charge of irrigation . . . it controls the water passages."[24] Its primary purpose is to facilitate the production and smooth dissemination of Qi and Fluids. It does this by "letting out," or "insuring free passage" of Qi, Fluids, or both in each of the three Heaters. In the Upper Heater it lets out the Defensive Qi from the Lung, insuring free passage between the skin and muscles throughout the body. In the Middle Heater it lets out the Nutritive Qi from the Stomach, insuring free flow to all of the Organs and through all of the channels. In the Lower Heater it lets out the body Fluids, insuring their free elimination from the Bladder.

The second view of the Triple Heater, as an "avenue of the Original Qi," comes from the Nan Jing. The author described the Triple Heater as "having a name, but no form,"[25] being only a collection of functions to disseminate Yuan Qi. This perspective considers the Triple Heater to be the means whereby the Original Qi of Ming Men is spread to the five Yin and six Yang Organs, and through the twelve channels, in order to provide the heat necessary to activate all of our physiological functions. This view also considers the end function of the Triple Heater to be the same as in the first view, that is, in facilitating digestion and the elimination of Fluids, although the means whereby this is accomplished are different. The Nan Jing states that the "Triple Heater is the avenue of food and drink, the beginning and end of Qi."[26] That the Triple Heater centers around the reception, transformation, transportation, and excretion of food and fluids is evidenced by the comments, "the Upper Heater controls receiving but not excreting," the Middle Heater controls "rotting and ripening of food and drink," and the Lower Heater controls "excreting but not receiving."[27]

The third view, common to both schools of thought, anatomically divides the body into three distinct Heaters, each with its own physiological functions. The Upper Heater consists of the area from the diaphragm upward, including the Heart, Lung, Heart Envelope, throat, and head. Its principle function is the even distribution of Defensive Qi and Fluids, in the form of a mist, from the Lung to all parts of the surface of the body. The Middle Heater, likened to a bubbling cauldron filled with foam, includes the region from the diaphragm to the umbilicus, and contains the Stomach, Spleen, and Gallbladder. Its functions include the digestion of food and drink and the transportation of the resultant Nutrient Qi to all parts of the body. The Lower Heater, described as a swamp or drainage ditch, includes the region from the umbilicus downward, and contains the Liver, Kidney, Large and Small Intestines, and Bladder. It serves to separate the clean and dirty parts of the digestate and to eliminate stool and urine. It should be noted that Western attempts to define Triple Heater function in terms of thermoregulation or control of the endocrine glands have no basis in traditional Chinese medicine.[28]

The Six Extraordinary (Curious) Yang Organs

In addition to the Yin and Yang Organs previously described, traditional Chinese medicine delineates six other Organs of which the *Su Wen* says, "Brain, Marrow, Bones, Blood Vessels, Gallbladder, and Uterus all store Yin Essences but have the shape of a Yang Organ (hollow); they store the Essence and do not excrete, therefore they are called Extraordinary (Curious) Yang Organs."[29] They are related to the Kidney, directly or indirectly, as they store some form of Yin Essence derived from Kidney Essence, Marrow, or Blood.

THE UTERUS

Also called "inside the lining" or the "red field," the Uterus is the most important of the Curious Organs. It regulates menstruation, conception, and pregnancy, and it is closely related to the Ren Mai and the Chong Mai, two Extraordinary Vessels that originate in Ming Men and are thus closely related to the Kidney. The Ren Mai provides the Uterus with Qi, while the Chong Mai provides it with Blood. Since both of these Extraordinary Vessels depend on Kidney Essence, when the Essence is abundant the Qi and Blood of the Uterus is adequate, and menstruation and pregnancy are normal. Because the Uterus is so intimately connected with the Blood, it has a functional relationship with the Heart, which governs the Blood; the Liver, which stores the Blood; and the Spleen, which controls the Blood. Failure of the Spleen to produce enough Blood or the Liver to store adequate Blood results in various dysfunctions of menstrual activity. Reproductive disorders are related to the Kidney Organ. Because the Chong Mai is also connected to the Stomach, Uterine upset can easily affect the Stomach, as happens with morning sickness during pregnancy. In men the Uterus is called "the room of Essence" and produces the sperm. It is closely related to the Du Mai and Kidney.

THE MARROW

Marrow, in the sense used here, should not be confused with the Western medical concept of bone marrow. Marrow, converted from Kidney Essence, is the precursor material for the Brain and spinal cord, as well as for the bone marrow. The *Su Wen* says, "The refined essence of food is changed into fat, it enters the bone cavities and fills the Brain with Marrow."[30]

THE BRAIN

The *Su Wen* calls the Brain "the Sea of Marrow, extending from the top of the head to the point Fengfu (GV16)."[31] The functions ascribed to it are very similar to the functions assigned by Western medicine and include sight, hearing, smell, touch, and intelligence. The Brain is under the control of the Kidney and Heart. Kidney Essence produces Marrow that fills up the Brain and spinal cord. Heart Blood nourishes the Brain. When Essence and Blood are abundant, Brain function is good.

THE BONES

The Bones are Yang Organs that store Marrow, by virtue of which they are controlled by the Kidney. The Kidney is therefore stimulated to speed bone healing.

THE BLOOD VESSELS

The Blood Vessels are considered Yang Organs that contain Blood. Since Blood is produced partly from the bone marrow derived from Kidney Essence, and partly from Food Qi that needs the Original Qi of the Kidney to transform into Blood, the Blood Vessels are also related to the Kidney.

THE GALLBLADDER

The Gallbladder is considered a Curious Organ because it stores bile, a pure substance. This is unlike the other Yang Organs that transform and digest but do not store. In all other regards the Gallbladder is considered a normal Yang Organ.

CHAPTER 4

ORIENTAL ANATOMY: MERIDIAN AND ACUPOINT THEORY

ENERGY FIELDS: THE SPHERE OF HEAVEN

Before the dawn of recorded history, Oriental physician-priests made an astounding discovery about the energetic nature of the human body. They discovered that the physical body is surrounded by a perceptible energy field that exhibits the precise condition of all of our internal organs and systems in real time. Characterized by the ancient Chinese as the Sphere of Heaven, this most subtle level of our being is comprised of the sum total of the various energy fields within our bodies. Part of the genius of Oriental medicine is the recognition of these fields and the subsequent development of treatment strategies to bring them into balance.

This basic human biofield was described by Chinese Daoists and Indian Ayurvedic physicians alike as the energy or astral body. Not usually perceptible to the normal senses, the energy body takes the shape of, and provides the motive force for, the gross physical body. I conjecture that this whole-body field is made up of the myriad interlocking electromagnetic fields of the entire pathway system in addition to the fields of the muscles and organs and their neurological control systems.

The biofield represents the most subtle range of therapeutic interaction available to the normal therapist, being affected as much by the intentions of the therapist and the therapist's own energy field as by the therapeutic manipulations employed. The sphere of interaction between the most physical part of the mind and the most subtle aspect of the body, the energy field has been the arena of hand-healers throughout history. The Chinese created many systems, generically called *qi kung*, for personal development of the energy body to enhance both healing and martial arts practices. Today this range of interaction is gaining credibility through the work of Delores Krieger and the therapeutic touch movement within the nursing profession. Other forms of energy-based healing in therapeutic massage and bodywork include the various forms of jin shin and reiki being practiced in the

Oriental bodywork community, as well as craniosacral therapy and polarity therapy currently practiced in the Western bodywork community.

MERIDIANS, CHANNELS, AND VESSELS: THE SPHERE OF MAN

Examining the body itself, the Chinese observed that the surface is covered by a complex network of energy-conducting pathways, which they characterized as the Sphere of Man. These pathways—called meridians, channels, or vessels according to their functions—also form branches that dive deep inside the body to pass through their related internal organs, infusing the fascial wrappings of that bowel or viscera, as well as that of the Element-related Organ with which they are associated in Oriental physiology. These internal meridians are frequently considered as the main trunks of the pathway complex. This is the functional mechanism that connects the Element-related organ/viscera pairs. I conjecture that the reflex sensations radiating from many trigger points follow these internal pathways. Interconnected Collateral Channels also connect one pathway to another, allowing the vital flow of Qi and Blood to pass from pathway to pathway in a fixed sequence each day. The recent archeological discovery of the *Han Ma-wang* (Burial mound silk books), medical texts predating the *Nei Jing*, shows that knowledge of the meridians predates recognition of the acupoints themselves.[1]

The meridian system is made up of several different kinds of pathways. The *jing-luo** are usually divided into two categories. The first category includes the twelve Organ meridians (Jing) and the eight Extraordinary Vessels (Qi Jing Ba Mai). The second category encompasses the Collateral Channels (Luo). We will cover the Extraordinary Vessels after the Collateral Channels.

Regular Meridians

The twelve Organ meridians and the Governor Vessel and Conception Vessel have been referred to as the Fourteen Regular Meridians since Hou Shou's fourteenth-century publication of the *Shi-si Jing Fa-hui* (Elaboration of the fourteen meridians).[2] The Governor Vessel (Du Mai) and Conception Vessel (Ren Mai) are included with the Organ meridians, as they alone among the Extraordinary Vessels have their own separate points and pathways; they are also included with the Organ meridians because of their profound involvement in Organ meridian function.

The Organ meridians each:

1. pertain to one of the internal Organ functions;
2. have their own unique set of superficial acupoints;
3. have major internal courses that connect them to one or more of the internal Organs;
4. have one or more minor Collateral Channels that connect them to other pathways.

Collateral Channels

The Collateral Channels are classified into three categories. The largest, called Collateral Connecting Channels, serve to interconnect the Element-related meridians, linking, for example, the Lung Meridian to the Large Intestine Meridian and the Large Intestine Meridian back to the Lung Meridian. There are fifteen Collateral Connecting Channels. In addition to linking the twelve Organ meridians, the Conception and Governor Vessels

---

* *Jing* means "to go through" or "a thread in a fabric"; *luo* means "something that connects or attaches" or "a net."

are also connected by this system. The Spleen, because of its primary role in producing and controlling the Blood, has two Collateral Channels.

The second category of Collateral Channels is comprised of the Superficial and Reticular Channels on the surface of the body. They serve to connect the flow of Qi and Blood from the regular meridians to all of the tissues of the body. They are the domain of the Defensive (Wei) Qi, the functional category the Chinese used in referring to both the cellular and the humoral components of the immune system. Changes in the energetic condition of the tissues underlying the skin profoundly affects the ability of both humoral antibodies and cellular defenders to rapidly respond to any crisis. Herein lies one of the mechanisms whereby BodyWork Shiatsu causes enhanced immune system response.

The third category pertains to the twelve Divergent Channels that help to enhance communication between the internal Organs and their superficial meridian extensions, as well as their Element-related meridians. This function differs from that of the Connecting Channels in that the Divergent Channels connect the internal Organs to the meridians, while the Connecting Channels connect meridian to meridian.

Finally, there are twelve cutaneous regions on the dermis and twelve tendino-muscle pathways in the myofascia. These are not actually distinct pathways but regions of skin and myofascia that are specifically affected by the pathways that course through them. The superficial myofascial regions that comprise the tendino-muscle channels associated with each of the regular meridians are one of the primary targets of Oriental bodywork. The condition of the myofascial tissues through which the energetic central core of the meridian passes are in a mutually interdependent relationship with the flow of Qi through the meridian. Changes in the tonus of the tendino-muscle channel will affect the energy flow in the meridians and vice versa. The muscle tests used in applied kinesiology to test the meridians are derived from these relationships.

The pathways are the "communication lines" of the body; they serve to carry Qi, Blood, and Fluids to all of its various parts. The *Nan Jing* states: "The pathways move Blood and Qi and insure the free flow of Yin and Yang, so that the body is properly nourished."[3] It is my experience that when palpated, meridians feel like very fine tubes of flowing energy. This flow of Qi is experienced proprioceptively as a fluidlike movement beneath the palpating fingers. Western physical science shows that energy flowing through a conductor behaves according to the same laws as fluids passing through a container. Depending on the degree of restriction or movement of the Qi, the tactile sensation ranges from intractably viscous and stuck to energetically fluid and free-flowing. Like electrical wires, the meridians are perceived as having a high-density solid energetic core with a surrounding field that diminishes in density and intensity as you move farther from the center.

A thorough understanding of the pathway system has great relevance in four areas: physiology, pathology, pattern identification, and treatment design.

Physiologically, the pathways serve the nutritive function of transporting Qi, Blood, and Fluids to all parts of the body. The pathways also serve as the lines of communication that link the various body parts into a unified whole.

Pathologically, the pathways represent the routes of entry for, and transmission of, pathogenic factors. This process is described in the *Su Wen*:

A pathogen settling in the body must first abide in the surface skin and body hair. If it resists expulsion, it will enter the Reticular Connecting Channels. If it continues to resist, it will enter the larger Connecting Channels. If it persists, it will enter the major meridians that communicate with the Organs in the inner body. When the pathogen spreads to the Stomach and Intestines, Yin and Yang are both affected and all the Organs suffer damage. This is the sequence by which pathogens entering the body through the surface skin and body hair eventually affect the five viscera.[4]

The interconnectedness of the internal Organs permits pathogenesis to spread from one Organ to another. Through this network the energetic balance of one Organ can affect the functions of another. Acupoints and pathways provide the physiological substrate for the manipulations that create balanced functioning between the Organs. The basic BodyWork Shiatsu treatment presented in part four works on the meridians to create and sustain dynamic homeostasis throughout the body.

Pattern identification and treatment design are two sides of one coin. By knowing the superficial course of the pathways and their internal interconnections, and by understanding the specific pathological conditions that arise when pathway function is disturbed, specific patterns of pathology can be identified. From this pattern recognition the appropriate acupoints and pathways can be identified and the proper treatment design formulated. Remediation of disease through pattern identification and treatment design is part of advanced BodyWork Shiatsu.

In Chinese medicine, treatment selection is always based on the specific presenting condition of the client. This differs radically from the Western medical approach of naming a disease and then offering a generic treatment to all persons suffering from that disease, regardless of their constitution or current condition. With the focus on treating the specific constellation of conditions presented at each session, treatments for specific disease states will vary not only from client to client, but also from treatment to treatment. This individualized, person-centered approach to therapy marks one major difference between Eastern and Western medicine.

Extraordinary Vessels

Representing an information control system that phylogenetically predates the development of the central nervous system, the Qi Jing Ba Mai (Extraordinary Vessels) begin to form coincident with conception. Starting with the first division of the fertilized ovum, this root energetic system carries the structural information that controls ontological development. Embryologically the formation of the first three Extraordinary Vessels (the Governing, Conception, and Penetrating Vessels) is coincident with the differentiation of the blastula into ectodermic, mesodermic, and endodermic layers.[5]

Developing prior to the central nervous system or the internal organs, the Extraordinary Vessels guide and determine the development of body structure. Beginning with conception, bioelectromagnetic fields are generated that control the placement of every molecule in the developing fetus. They guide and direct the growth and relationship of all aspects of our structure. Forming as fields of interaction between the bioelectromagnetic energies of the human body and the magnetosphere of the Earth, the Qi Jing Ba Mai also perform the function of reservoirs, acting to absorb excess energy from the regular pathway system when Qi overflows. The *Nan Jing* says: "If the twelve meridians are full to overflowing, this fullness spills over into the eight Extraordinary Vessels, never to return."[6]

The earliest references to the Extraordinary Vessels are found in the *Nei Jing*. The term translated as "Extraordinary," Qi, generally refers to something exceptional, unusual, strange, rare, or wonderful. The oldest usage of this term occurs in reference to an unusually shaped or deformed body, someone hunched over, sloping to one side or handicapped by a physical deformity.[7] The author of the *Nan Jing* simplified and systematized the Extraordinary Vessels pathway descriptions and added concise symptomatologies. Here we also find the first clearly developed energetic theories concerning the Extraordinary Vessels, differentiating them from Five Element and Regular Meridian energetics.

The Extraordinary Vessels are controlled by master points located on the regular meridians and treated in paired sets, the sets being characterized by common relationships that further explain the nature of their interaction. These points, pairings, and relationships are:

Chong Mai (Sp4)↔Yin Wei Mai (HE6)
(Father and Mother)
Ren Mai (Lu7)↔Yin Qiao Mai (Ki6)
(Master and Guest)
Dai Mai (Gb41)↔Yang Wei Mai (TH5)
(Male and Female)
Du Mai (SI3)↔Yang Qiao Mai (Bl62)
(Husband and Wife)

The *Nan Jing* theorizes an intersection between the macrocosm and microcosm at the energetic, and physical, center of the body, "the moving Qi between the kidneys," variously identified as Ming Men, the "Small Heart," and Qihai Dan tien. The *Nan Jing* describes this region as, "The root of the twelve meridians, fundamental to the five yin and six yang organs; the source of the Triple Heater, the Gate of Breathing; the source of the vital Qi."[8] The author of the *Nan Jing*, following Daoist thought, saw two distinct yet related lines of manifestation from ultimate formlessness into form. Both originate at this central axis of the intersection of the Heaven↔Human↔Earth triad.

Wu Chi, the Great Ultimate, begins its descent into form at the level of no form, the Dao. Matsumoto and Birch liken the state of no form to David Bohm's concept of "an implicate order, a vast ocean of energy in space, a vast universal hidden matrix."[9] According to the Daoists, this universal matrix is the precursor of matter: "Its child is light, its grandchild is water. All is created from No Form."[10] The relationship to the modern concepts of quantum physics regarding the primacy of energy over matter are obvious. The separation becomes complete as the Dao separates into Yin and Yang. The One becomes Two.

From here creation follows two different pathways. In the most familiar line of manifestation the two become three: the Three Heaters. The Triple Heaters divide to become the six great energies: Tai Yang, Shao Yang, Yang Ming, Tai Yin, Shao Yin, and Jue Yin. These six energies form the basis of Qi circulation through the regular meridians in the Nutrient Cycle. In this cycle, the Qi flows up and down meridian pairs according to their great energy quality during each eight-hour period of the day. Thus, Qi flows through the Tai Yin and Yang Ming meridians on the anterior surface of the body from 3 A.M. to 11 A.M.; through the Shao Yin and Tai Yang meridians on the posterior portion of the body from 11 A.M. to 7 P.M.; and through the Shao Yang and Jue Yin meridians on the midline of the body from 7 P.M. to 3 A.M. These great energy pathways are then further divided into the twelve Organ meridians. In the other line of manifestation, the two becomes the four, the divisions of the body, which in turn become the eight, the eight Extraordinary Vessels.[11] These lines of manifestation are shown in figure 4.1.

Because they represent the manifestation of the root energetic pattern that determines our structure, the Extraordinary Vessels are predominantly used for the correction of structural imbalances.[12] Their prefetal manifestation seems to indi-

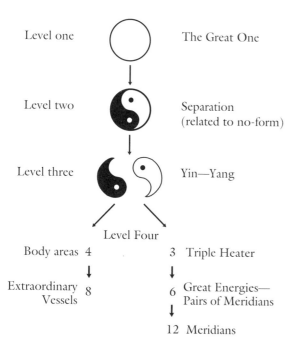

Level one — The Great One

Level two — Separation (related to no-form)

Level three — Yin—Yang

Level Four

Body areas 4   3 Triple Heater

Extraordinary Vessels 8   6 Great Energies— Pairs of Meridians

12 Meridians

Fig. 4.1. Development of the Twelve Meridians and the Eight Extraordinary Vessels

cate their existence more as fields of bio-electromagnetism than discrete pathways of Qi flow. This correlates clearly with the ancient description of the Qi Jing Ba Mai as "oceans" of energy. The existence of the Extraordinary Vessels as fields of force rather than pathways of Qi also explains their primary relationship with the bio-rhythmic fluctuations of the Earth's geomagnetic field as described in the *Nan Jing* and other source texts.[13] As electromagnetic fields, these "oceans" are arenas where energetic information from any one field interacts with and feeds back into each of the other participants in a general field effect.

Structure and function are never separate from each other but rather are different views of one primary event differentiated only in terms of time and energy.[14] One way to view the relationship between the Extraordinary Vessels and the regular pathways is to see the Heaven↔Human↔Earth triad in terms of energy, function, and structure (fig. 4.2). Energy, the first manifestation of formlessness into

form, embodies the archetype of Heaven: formless, mutable, creative, Yang. Structure, the quintessential concretization of Earth, is archetypal Yin. The essence of organic human life, function is the by-product of this ultimate Yin-Yang interaction.

While the above discussion places the Extraordinary Vessel field network in a different, more primordial, relationship to human structure than the jing-luo, the regular pathways and the Extraordinary Vessels still constantly interact and affect each other. After all, three of the Extraordinary Vessels are in primary relationship with the regular pathway system. The Ren Mai is called "the ocean of the Yin," the Du Mai is the "the ocean of the Yang," and the Chong Mai is "the ocean of the twelve meridians, the five Yin and six Yang Organs, and the ocean of the Blood." Structural information and functional information always exist side by side.

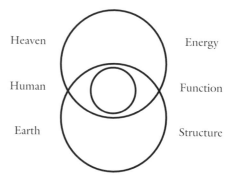

Heaven   Energy

Human   Function

Earth   Structure

Fig. 4.2. Energy↔Function↔Structure Continuum

THE ACUPOINTS: THE SPHERE OF EARTH

The acupoint system, designated the Sphere of Earth by the Chinese, is a superset of all of the possible energetic loci that can be found on the surface of the human body. An energetic locus is a point of very concentrated energy, existent at or just below the surface of the body, that acts as a focus for specific structural, biological, and energetic events.

There are more than one thousand such loci, called acupoints, on the body. Seven hundred twenty of these lie on the Organ meridians; another approximately three hundred extra points are found on nonmeridian locations.

Manipulation of the acupoints creates local and distant energetic effects, as well as neurological, circulatory, and myofascial effects. Manipulation of an acupoint can directly affect the function of entire meridians or the internal Organs associated with those meridians. Manipulation can intensify or diminish the activities of specific nerves or control entire segments of the nervous system. Manipulation can also have general effects on the organism as a whole.

Due to the variety of different nerve receptors at each acupoint, many different forms of stimulation or sedation are possible, depending on the therapeutic techniques employed. I believe this rich neural field is the physiological mechanism underlying the effectiveness of the many techniques employed to influence the energetic system.

One measure of the subtlety of Oriental medicine is the recognition that events taking place at the surface of the body can profoundly affect internal functions and vice versa. There is a maxim in Oriental therapy that states, "Evaluation is treatment," recognizing that the very act of touching affects the involved reflection of internal conditions. This reciprocal feedback relationship appears to be mediated by the autonomic nervous system and allows for bidirectional communication between the surface of the body and the internal Organ systems and their functions. The thoraco-lumbar (Shu/Yu) Associated points and the abdomino-thoracic (Mu/Bo) Alarm points are representative of this. They display the reflexes for the Organ-related functions of the sympathetic and parasympathetic nervous systems respectively.[15]

The Element or Command points are a series of points located between the fingertips and elbows or toe tips and knees on each meridian. These points have been given different designations and accorded various functions in the classics. The oldest categorization, from the *Nei Jing*, describes how the Qi starts out most superficially at the fingertips or toe tips and gradually broadens and deepens as it moves toward the elbows and knees. This is the same for all of the meridians, whether Yin or Yang. In this framework the most distal point is likened to a well, where the Qi flows out, the second point to a spring, where it slips and glides, the third to a stream, where it pours, the fourth to a river, where it moves freely, and the fifth to a sea, where the Qi enters deeply into the body. Because the Qi is so superficial in the extremities and because it is here that the polarity changes from Yin to Yang and back, these points present a very large repertoire of functions.

The best known of these functions, first elucidated in the *Nan Jing*, are the Element points. Thus, each meridian has a point corresponding to each of the five Elements; these points are used to correct the balance of both Organs and meridians using the Creation and Control cycles of Five Element theory. Other Command points include the Source point, which receives the Source Qi from the dan tien as distributed to each of the meridians by the Triple Heater in the Nutrient Cycle (described in the next section). The Connecting points open channels between the Element-related meridians that allow them to stay in balance. For example, if the Lung is in Excess and the Large Intestine Deficient, the connecting points would allow them to balance each other out. The Cleft points are spots where Qi gets stuck in acute disorders and are used to relieve pain in those circumstances. Horary points become active during the two-hour period of maximum activity of each meridian and are used to enhance the effectiveness of treatment given at the those times.

The Master points for the Extraordinary Vessels, all located on acupoints of the regular meridians, seem to operate by changing the intensity of the basic biofields that keep our structural integrity intact. The addition or subtraction of energy generated by finger pressure to the precise locus of the biofields that control these functions is sufficient to alter the strength of these biofields. This changes the threshold of response and thus the functioning of the entire system being treated.[16]

The phenomenon of trigger points, classically called Ah Shi ("That's it!") points, works through an entirely different mechanism. These points are the focus of noxious irritation in the soft tissues due to imbalanced structure, strain or sprain, toxicity, or trauma. The pain-spasm-pain cycle that characterizes trigger points is maintained reflexively in the internuncial pool of the spinal cord, without the need for higher medullary or cortical intervention. Pain radiating from these points may travel along the meridians (especially their internal branches), along various nerves, or along the planes of myofascia, causing irritation at specific points that may or may not correspond to traditional acupoints. They frequently manifest at the locations indicated for the nonmeridian Special points, but may manifest anywhere on the body.

Acupoints change their size and relative location depending on the intensity of the imbalance they reflect. Exact acupoint location will always depend on the alignment of the body with its biofield, and considerable variation is possible. The acupoint itself can vary in size at any given time from not physically present to the size of a quarter. Ah Shi points or active Shu/Yu point reflexes can extend over a considerable area, although reactivity is directly proportional to the distance from the exact center of the energetic locus of the acupoint.

THE COURSE OF THE MERIDIANS

The Oriental anatomical position differs from the Western anatomical position in that the hands are raised over the head, with the palms facing forward (fig. 4.3). This position allows for uniformity in describing the direction of flow of the meridians. The pathways on the anterior aspect of the body are Yin; those on the posterior surface are Yang. (If you visualize a person on hands and knees, the pathways facing the Earth are Yin and those facing the sun are Yang.)

In this anatomical position the Yang meridians always descend from Heaven to Earth, and the Yin pathways always rise from Earth to Heaven. This is why we follow the convention of describing the Yin pathways of the arms as "ascending" the arm even though in the Western anatomical position they seem to "descend" from the torso to the fingertips.

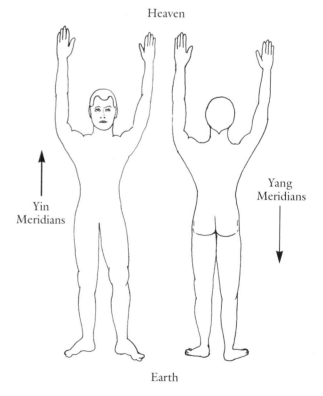

Fig. 4.3. Oriental Anatomical Position

The Nutrient Cycle

Beginning with the Lung meridian, which is Yin in nature and originates on the torso, the Nutritive Qi in the body flows in a tidal pattern from Yin meridian to Yang meridian to Yin meridian to Yang meridian, continuing in this rhythm as it travels a full circuit through the pairs of Element-related pathways once every twenty-four hours. Ascending the Yin pathways of the arms from torso to fingertips, the energy flow undergoes a polar transformation into its opposite quality and then descends the coupled Yang pathway of the arm to the face. There it transfers to the Yang pathway of the legs and follows its course to the toes, where it once again transforms into its opposite and ascends the coupled Yin meridian of the legs. The Qi then returns to the torso, and the cycle begins all over again.

This remarkable transformation in the quality of the energy flowing through the meridians is what sets the stage for the therapeutic response elicited by Oriental manipulation techniques. Specifically, it is at the points of transformation, at the extremities, where Yin transmutes to Yang and vice versa, that the appropriate and timely application of the various techniques of Oriental medicine can be most effective. Influencing the course and nature of the energy flow, these manipulations can serve to recreate the harmonious energetic balance between the Organ pathways, thus allowing the self-healing capabilities of the body to emerge.

Knowing when maximum energy flows through each pathway is of diagnostic value, since symptoms that consistently present at a regular time are indicative of the Organ-pathway complex involved in the imbalance. Table 4.1 shows the timing and order of the cyclic flow of Nutritive Qi throughout the body. Each two-hour period activates special points, called Horary points, in each pathway. Treatment of these points during their active phase increases the effectiveness of Organ-pathway treatment.

TABLE 4.1

The Timing and Order of Nutrient Cycle Flow

(Note: Times shown are Standard time.)

Lung Meridian of Hand—Tai Yin	From torso to fingertip	3 A.M.–5 A.M.
Large Intestine Meridian of Hand—Yang Ming	From fingertip to face	5 A.M.–7 A.M.
Stomach Meridian of Foot—Yang Ming	From face to toe	7 A.M.–9 A.M.
Spleen/Pancreas Meridian of Foot—Tai Yin	From toe to torso	9 A.M.–11 A.M.
Heart Meridian of Hand—Shao Yin	From torso to fingertip	11 A.M.–1 P.M.
Small Intestine Meridian of Hand—Tai Yang	From fingertip to face	1 P.M.–3 P.M.
Bladder Meridian of Foot—Tai Yang	From face to toe	3 P.M.–5 P.M.
Kidney Meridian of Foot—Shao Yin	From foot to torso	5 P.M.–7 P.M.
Heart Envelope Meridian of Hand—Jue Yin	From torso to fingertip	7 P.M.–9 P.M.
Triple Heater Meridian of Hand—Shao Yang	From fingertip to face	9 P.M.–11 P.M.
Gallbladder Meridian of Foot—Shao Yang	From face to toe	11 P.M.–1 A.M.
Liver Meridian of Foot—Jue Yin	From foot to torso	1 A.M.–3 A.M.

The following pages describe the muscular and tendinous landmarks traversed by the superficial course of the meridians. The external pathway of the Governor and Conception Vessels are included with the Organ meridians.

The effectiveness of both diagnosis and treatment using the meridian system depends on the accuracy with which this system is accessed. A precise knowledge of the Organ relationships to tender points or areas is requisite for accurate evaluation of palpatory findings. And while the tendino-muscle channels are relatively broad and therefore somewhat forgiving of inaccurate treatment locations, precise finger placement yields infinitely better results. Though not totally applicable to entry-level treatment, a precise knowledge of the meridian system is absolutely required for continued growth as a BodyWork Shiatsu practitioner. The following charts should be referred to repeatedly as you learn the treatments offered in this book. (**Note:** In the following discussions the term *ungual* refers to the superior border of the fingernail.)

Lung Meridian

The Lung Meridian (fig. 4.4) begins 1 inch below the midpoint of the clavicle, in the first intercostal space directly below the infraclavicular fossa. It ascends to the inferior edge of the clavicle, turns laterally to the edge of the deltoid, and descends the shoulder along the delto-pectoral groove. The pathway continues to descend the arm along the radial edge of the biceps brachii to the radial edge of the biceps brachii tendon at the transverse cubital crease.

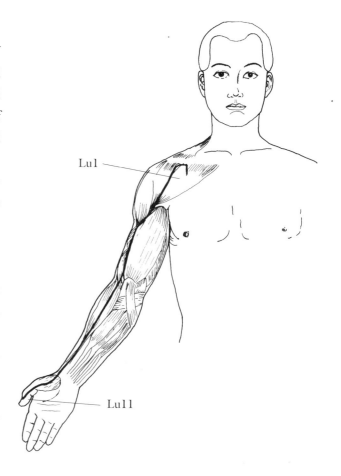

Fig. 4.4. *Lung Meridian*

The pathway descends the radial aspect of the anterior forearm between the brachioradialis and the flexor carpi radialis until it crosses the brachioradialis tendon 1½ inches proximal to the transverse wrist crease, where it continues to the crease between the brachioradialis tendon and the head of the radius.

The pathway continues distally through the thenar eminence between the abductor pollicis and the opponens pollicis to the first metacarpal bone. It follows the skin color change line to end ¹⁄₁₀ inch proximal to the radial ungual margin of the thumb.

Large Intestine Meridian

The Large Intestine Meridian (fig. 4.5) begins $\frac{1}{10}$ inch proximal to the radial ungual margin of the index finger, ascends the skin color change line of the index finger to pass between the first dorsal interosseous muscle and the abductor pollicis brevis, then crosses the dorsal wrist crease between the tendons of the extensor pollicis longus and extensor pollicis brevis.

The pathway ascends the radial aspect of the posterior forearm along the radial edge of the extensor carpi radialis brevis to the midpoint between the radial edge of the transverse cubital crease and the lateral epicondyle of the humerus.

Ascending the arm along the lateral intermuscular septum, the pathway continues on the lateral edge of the triceps brachii, passing to the acromion between the anterior and medial heads of the deltoid.

The pathway then runs medially along the anterior aspect of the trapezius and returns to the lateral border of the sternocleidomastoid ascending up the neck. It then crosses the digastricus and the buccinator and passes across the upper lip. The pathway ends at the lateral edge of the opposite nostril, even with the base of the ala nasi.

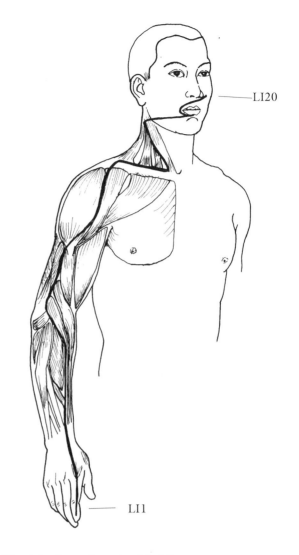

Fig. 4.5. *Large Intestine Meridian*

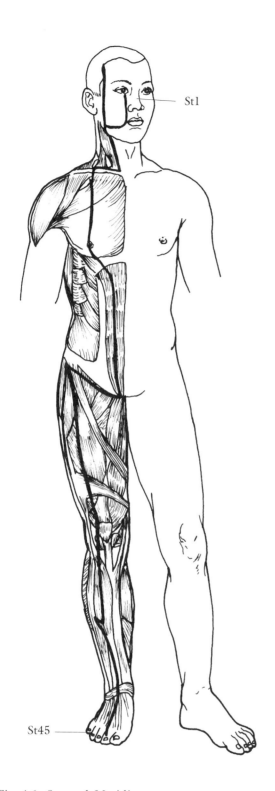

St1

St45

Fig. 4.6. Stomach Meridian

Stomach Meridian

The Stomach meridian (fig. 4.6) begins midorbitally in the orbicularis oculi and descends the cheek in a straight line to the orbicularis oris, 1/4 inch lateral to the edge of the mouth. It then curves laterally around the masseter and ascends the side of the face, through the mandibular condyle, to end in the galea aponeurotica, 1/2 inch above the original hairline.

A pathway branches at the masseter, passing through the digastricus and descending the throat along the anterior border of the sternocleidomastoid. At the clavicle the pathway runs laterally through the platysma along the superior border of the clavicle, crossing the clavicle and descending through the pectoralis major, in the mamillary line, to the fifth intercostal space. Here the pathway turns medio-inferior, to course bilaterally through the center of the rectus abdominis muscles from the seventh intercostal space to the superior edge of the pubic tubercle.

The pathway then turns latero-inferior, passing between the insertions of the sartorius and the tensor fascia latae, to run down the lateral edge of the rectus femoris to the lateral edge of the patella. It then descends the leg through the tibialis anterior. At the midpoint of the leg the pathway shifts 1 inch lateral to course down the extensor digitorum longus, to the middle of the ankle crease. The pathway then runs between the second and third metatarsals to end at the lateral ungual margin of the second toe.

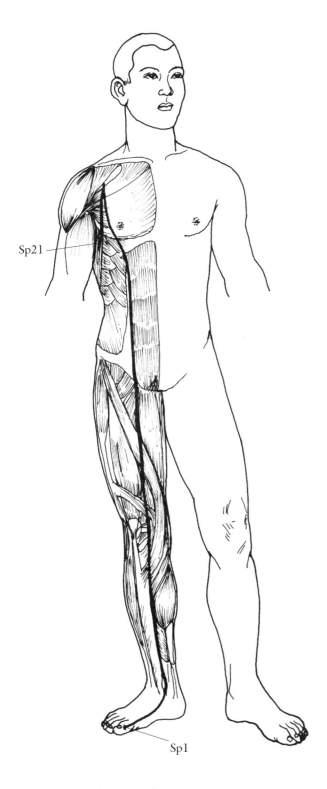

Sp21

Sp1

Fig. 4.7. Spleen Meridian

Spleen Meridian

The Spleen Meridian (fig. 4.7) begins $\frac{1}{10}$ inch proximal to the medial ungual margin of the big toe and runs up the skin color change line on the inside of the foot; it then passes in front of the medial malleolus and ascends the leg along the posterior border of the tibia.

Passing the medial border of the patella, the pathway ascends the thigh along the vastus medialis and, crossing over the sartorius, follows the adductor longus up to the femoral triangle. Passing through the iliacus, it ascends the torso along the lateral border of the rectus abdominis.

At the costal margin the pathway turns supero-lateral to ascend 2 inches lateral to the mamillary line, in the intercostal muscles at the lateral margin of the pectoralis, up to the second intercostal space. There it turns sharply infero-lateral, contouring the serratus anterior, to end in the seventh intercostal space in the midaxillary line.

Heart Meridian

The Heart Meridian (fig. 4.8) begins in the center of the axilla, at the latero-inferior margin of the pectoralis major. It descends the arm along the humeral groove, medial to the biceps brachii, to the midpoint between the cubital crease and the medial epicondyle of the humerus.

The pathway descends the medial aspect of the inside of the forearm between the flexor carpi ulnaris and the flexor digitorum superficialis to the transverse wrist crease. There it passes the palm between the fourth and fifth metacarpals, running along the skin color change line of the little finger to end $1/10$ inch proximal to the radial ungual margin of the fifth finger.

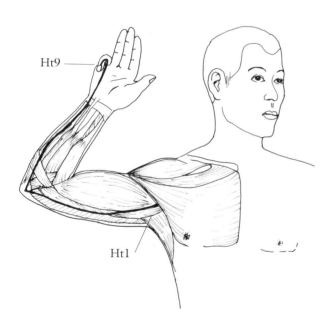

Fig. 4.8. Heart Meridian

Small Intestine Meridian

The Small Intestine Meridian (fig. 4.9) begins $1/10$ inch proximal to the ulnar ungual margin of the fifth finger, ascending the skin color change line of the ulnar aspect of the hand to the hollow between

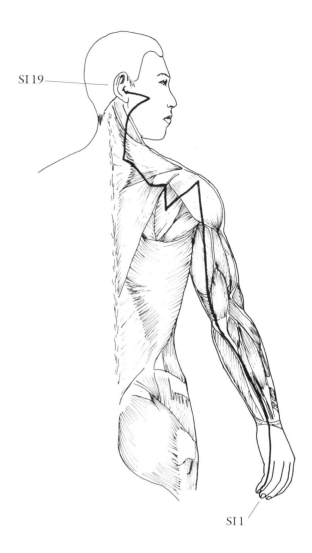

Fig. 4.9. Small Intestine Meridian

the pisiform bone and the styloid process of the ulna.

The pathway then ascends the forearm along the dorsal edge of the ulna to the midpoint between the olecranon process (the "funny bone") and the medial epicondyle of the humerus. The pathway continues by ascending the upper arm along the medial head of the triceps brachii, running to the inferior margin of the scapular spine in the posterior head of the deltoid.

The pathway zigzags over the scapula, pointing in the center of the infraspinatus, the center of the supraspinatus, and the origin of the levator scapulae. It then contours the levator scapulae to ascend the neck between the scalene muscles, and to the point between the angle of the mandible and the sternocleidomastoid.

The pathway passes over the masseter and buccinator to the point on the inferior border of the zygoma directly below the outer canthus of the eye, then turns lateral to end just anterior to the tragus of the ear.

Bladder Meridian

The Bladder Meridian (fig. 4.10) begins at the medial canthus of the eye and ascends the forehead in a vertical line to the natural hairline. Moving laterally ½ inch, the pathway contours the cranium through the frontal, parietal, and occipital bones to the lateral margin of the insertion of the superior head of the trapezius, between C1 and C2. Here the pathway splits into two branches.

The Bladder 1 (Bl1) pathway descends the dorsal surface of the erector spinae muscle group, 1 ½ inches lateral to the spinous processes. At the level of the sacral hiatus the pathway zigs back up to the top of the sacrum, then descends the sacrum through the foramina to the level of the coccyx. Slanting down to the midline of the posterior thigh, it descends between the hamstrings to the musculo-tendinous junction of the biceps femoris, following the medial edge of that tendon to the crease of the knee. There it turns medially, to end at the center of the popliteal fossa.

The Bl2 pathway begins at the insertion of the superior head of the trapezius and descends the lateral border of that muscle to the cervico-thoracic juncture. From there it descends the lateral border of the erector spinae muscle mass, 3 inches from the spinous processes, traveling down to the musculo-tendinous juncture of the gluteus maximus, at the

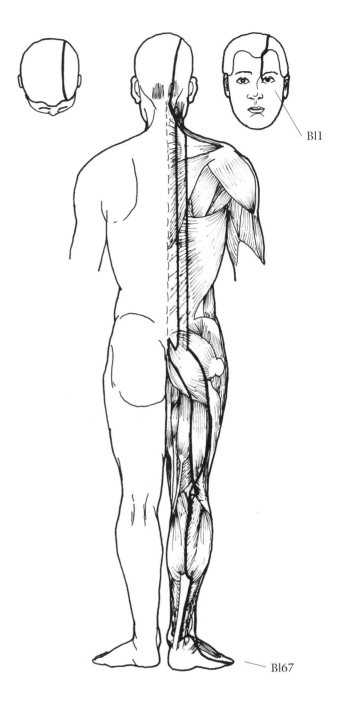

Fig. 4.10. Bladder Meridian

level of the sacral apex and overlying the inferior border of the piriformis.

The pathway continues its descent, contouring the gluteus maximus, and passes to the posterior thigh along the lateral border of the muscle belly of the biceps femoris. The pathway then veers to the posterior midline where it rejoins the first branch in the center of the popliteal fossa. From here the pathway has a single course. The pathway descends the posterior midline of the leg between the heads of the gastrocnemius. At the inferior border of the lateral head it turns to travel down the lateral margin of the Achilles tendon to the calcaneus. The pathway turns latero-superior to a point below the lateral malleolus. Then it follows the skin color change line to end $1/10$ inch proximal to the lateral ungual margin of the fifth toe.

Kidney Meridian

The Kidney Meridian (fig. 4.11) begins in the center of the sole of the foot, posterior to and between the heads of the first and second metatarsals, and runs supero-medially across the navicular tuberosity to the bottom of the medial malleolus. Here the pathway circles the medial side of the calcaneus, ascends 2 inches up the Achilles tendon, then jogs $1/2$ inch anterior to the border of the tibia, and ascends the soleus and medial head of the gastrocnemius, continuing to the lateral border of the tendon of the semitendinosus at the crease of the knee.

The pathway ascends the thigh along the medial border of the semitendinosus to the groin. After coursing internally through the pelvis, it becomes superficial at the superior border of the pubic ramus, at the medial margin of the muscle belly of the rectus abdominis.

The pathway then moves up the inside edge of the rectus abdominis to a point 6 inches above the umbilicus, where it slants latero-superior to the costochondral margin of the sternum at the fifth intercostal space. Then it ascends the lateral border of the sternum to end at the inferior border of the clavicle.

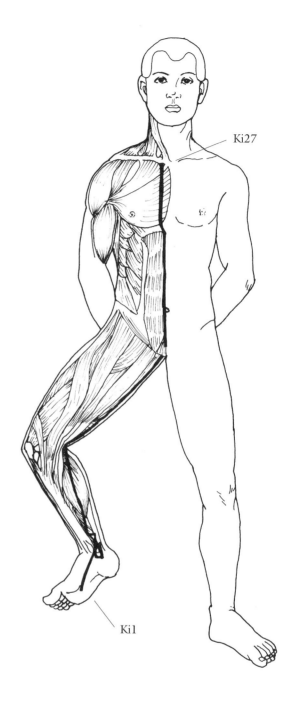

Fig. 4.11. Kidney Meridian

Triple Heater Meridian

The Triple Heater Meridian (fig. 4.13) begins $\frac{1}{10}$ inch proximal to the ulnar ungual margin of the ring finger and crosses the dorsal surface of the hand to the wrist crease between the tendons of the extensor digitorum and the extensor digiti minimi.

The pathway then ascends the dorsal midline of the forearm along the ulnar border of the extensor digitorum longus, pointing 3 inches proximal to the wrist crease, then 1 inch directly lateral, before returning to the extensor digitorum longus margin to a point 1 inch above the olecranon process, in

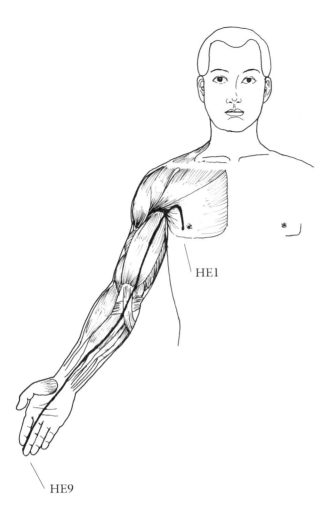

Fig. 4.12. Heart Envelope Meridian

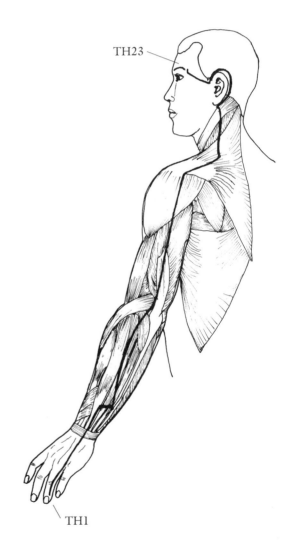

Fig. 4.13. Triple Heater Meridian

Heart Envelope Meridian

The Heart Envelope Meridian (fig. 4.12) begins in the pectoralis major, overlying the fourth intercostal space, 1 inch lateral to the nipple. Contouring the pectoralis insertion, it descends the center of the anterior arm between the heads of the biceps brachii, to point on the ulnar side of the biceps brachii tendon at the cubital crease.

The pathway descends the anterior midline of the forearm to the wrist crease between the palmaris longus and the flexor carpi radialis. It then crosses the palm between the second and third metacarpals, ending $\frac{1}{10}$ inch proximal to the radial ungual margin of the middle finger.

the tendon of the triceps brachii. It continues up the posterior midline of the arm along the long head of the triceps brachii to the postero-inferior border of the acromion process, between the middle and posterior heads of the deltoid, then passes medially along the supraspinatous fossa to the insertion of the levator scapulae, and over the medial trapezius to the back of the neck.

The pathway travels up the neck along the lateral border of the posterior scalene muscles to a point between the mastoid process and the mandibular angle. It then contours the hairline around the ear to the tuberculum supratragicum, turning medio-superior to end at the zygomatico-frontal suture, lateral to the edge of the eyebrow.

Gallbladder Meridian

The Gallbladder Meridian (fig. 4.14), which begins ½ inch lateral to the outer canthus of the eye, contours the inferior border of the zygomatic arch to a point in front of the intertragic notch. It first turns superior to a point at the temporo-parietal suture, then turns infero-lateral through the temporal fossa within the hairline to a point just above the apex of the ear. Now the pathway curves around the ear, about 1½ inches from the auricle, through the temporal fossa to the insertion of the sternocleidomastoid, inferior to the mastoid process. The pathway returns through the temporalis insertions on the occiput, parietal, and frontal bones to a point in the supercilliary arch, 1 inch above the center of the eyebrow. It recurves posteriorly, coursing along the frontal, parietal, and occipital eminences to a point between the occipital tuberosity and the mastoid process.

The pathway descends the neck along the antero-lateral margin of the superior head of the trapezius. It then passes laterally along the top of the medial head of the trapezius to the acromion. Descending along the delto-pectoral groove, fol-

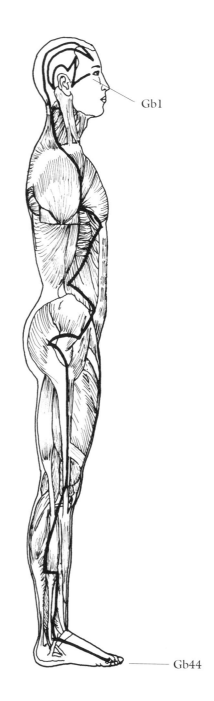

Fig. 4.14. Gallbladder Meridian

lowing the curve of the serratus anterior, the pathway points 3 inches below the axilla, in the fifth intercostal space, on the lateral midline. Now the pathway curves antero-inferior, to point in the mamillary line in the seventh intercostal space; it then curves postero-inferior, following the costal arch, to point at the tip of the twelfth rib.

The pathway continues in an antero-inferior curve, running through the abdominal aponeuroses and contouring the curve of the ilium to point just medial to the anterior superior iliac spine (ASIS). It then continues laterally, to a point on the musculo-tendinous border of the gluteus maximus, overlying the piriformis.

From here the pathway descends the lateral midline of the thigh and leg, coursing through the tensor fascia latae and the peroneal muscles overlying the fibula, veering anterior midway down the leg and continuing to a point antero-inferior to the lateral malleolus. Passing between the fourth and fifth metatarsals, the pathway ends $\frac{1}{10}$ inch proximal to the lateral ungual margin of the fourth toe.

Liver Meridian

The Liver Meridian (fig. 4.15) begins $\frac{1}{10}$ inch proximal to the lateral ungual margin of the large toe and ascends the dorsum of the foot between the first and second metatarsals, pointing 1 inch distal to the medial malleolus at the medial edge of the tibialis anterior tendon. Passing in front of the malleolus, the pathway ascends the posterior border of the tibia for half the length of the leg. It then passes posterior to the Spleen pathway, and coursing through the medial aspect of the medial head of the gastrocnemius, crosses the knee at the medial edge of the knee crease.

The pathway ascends the thigh along the posterior border of the vastus medialis to the inguinal fossa. It then curves around the genitals and ascends the torso along the curve of the abdominal aponeurosis to a point at the tip of the eleventh rib. It continues to arc around the supero-medial portion of the aponeurosis, to end at the medial edge of the sixth intercostal space.

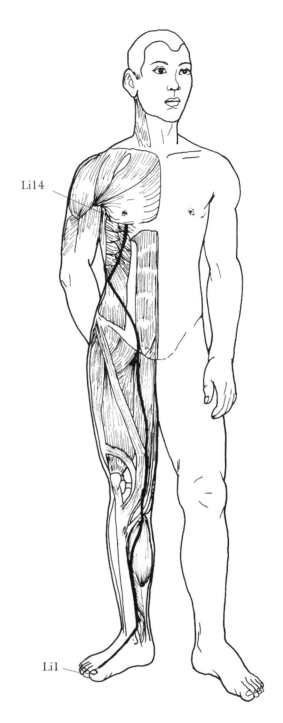

Fig. 4.15. Liver Meridian

Governor Vessel (Du Mai)

The Governor Vessel (fig. 4.16) begins in the anococcygeal ligament, just anterior to the tip of the coccyx. It ascends the dorsal midline through the center of the spinous processes; then it bisects the cranium, passing through the sagittal suture and curving over the forehead. Finally it descends the nasal septum, bisects the philtrum, and curls under the upper lip to end at the labial frenulum.

Conception Vessel (Ren Mai)

The Conception Vessel (fig. 4.17) begins in the central perineal tendon and ascends the ventral midline, bisecting the pubic symphysis and coursing up the linea alba. Passing through the center line of the sternum, the throat, and the mandibular suture, the pathway ends in the center of the mentolabial groove under the lower lip.

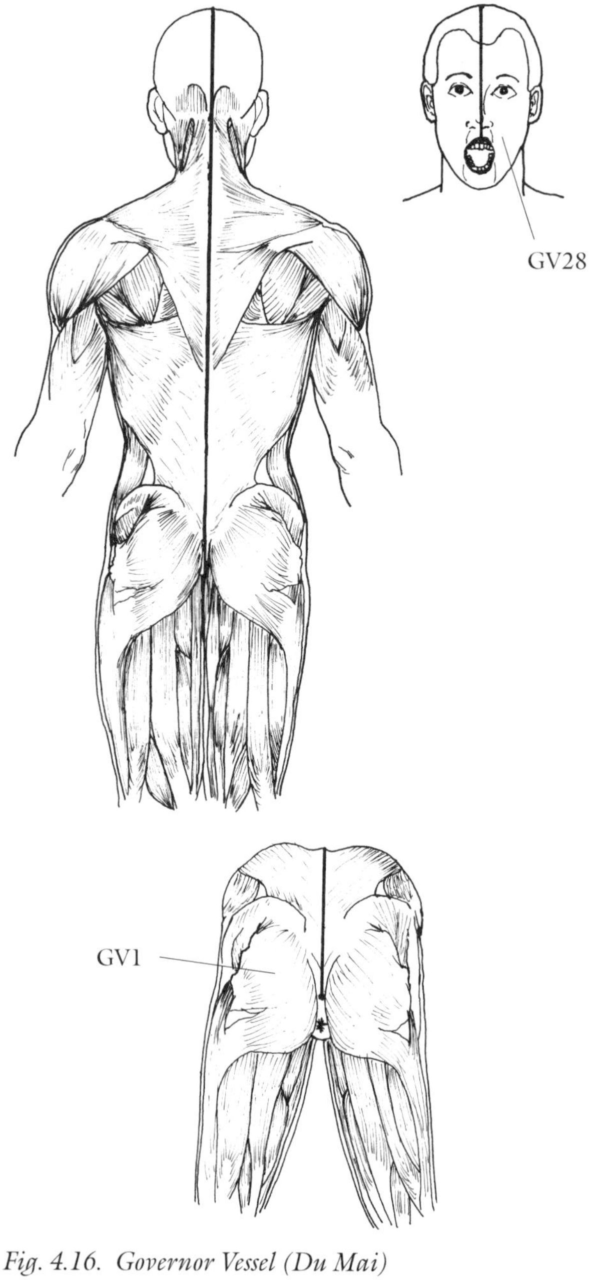

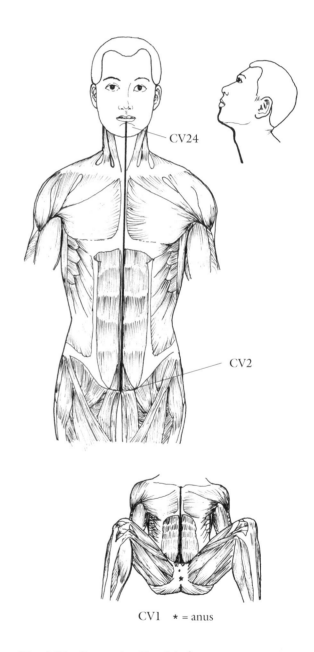

GV28

GV1

CV24

CV2

CV1   ⋆ = anus

Fig. 4.16. Governor Vessel (Du Mai)

Fig. 4.17. Conception Vessel (Ren Mai)

CHAPTER 5

ORIENTAL ASSESSMENT AND DIAGNOSIS

THE CAUSES OF DISEASE

Developing within the cultural conditions of ancient China, considerations of disease pathogenesis mirrored the Chinese philosophical views of the relationship of the human to the cosmos. Illness was not seen as an isolated set of symptoms affecting individual body parts or organs, nor as the simple effect of microbial invasion, but rather as the interaction between external meteorological conditions, internal emotional states, lifestyle habits, and attacks by pestilential factors, all countered by the natural immune functions of the body and the preexisting harmony of the Organs and emotions.

The Chinese saw an interaction between complementary opposites in all things. In the realm of health, this play takes place in the balance between Yin and Yang, Blood and Qi, and the Organs and meridians. When the harmony between the person and the environment is disrupted, external, internal, or lifestyle imbalances may manifest as disease. If the body's vital immune function is strong enough, Nutritive Qi and Defensive Qi, combined

to form Correct Qi (Zheng Qi), can protect against the invasion of external pathogenic Qi. Internal causes represent imbalances between the emotions and Organs, disturbing the body's Yin and Yang. The *Ling Shu* says: "When Yin is calm, and Yang is sound, the spirit is undisturbed."[1] The nineteenth-century European tradition of natural hygiene most closely duplicates this worldview and has given birth to the modern Western medical approach called ecological medicine.

External Causes

The external factors that cause disease relate to meteorological conditions and their timing and intensity, as well as hereditary and lifestyle habits that predispose us to be vulnerable to one factor or another. Microbial pathogens are also considered as external factors. The natural adaptive response of the human body to environmental changes normally protects us from harm. The shift of seasons, from winter to spring, for example, causes a natural opening up to the environment. The entire natural world undergoes this change. Plants bud, animals come out of hibernation, and Correct Qi flows to the surface, preparing us to interact openly with the environment after the rest and renewal of winter. It is only when this normal adaptive function fails to respond appropriately to the environment that seasonal conditions become environmental excesses. The *Su Wen* states: "Though there may be wind, rain, cold, or heat, without depletion and emptiness, pathogens alone cannot harm the body. The ability to stand up to raging winds and sudden storms without becoming ill indicates that there is no lack of Qi allowing harm to the health."[2]

It is important to note that the conditions described indicate internal responses and manifestations within the body as well as meteorological phenomena in the environment. The environmental excesses first mentioned in the *Nei Jing* are Wind, Cold, Heat, Damp, Summer Heat, and Dryness. Pestilential Qi was first recognized as an External Excess in the fourteenth century C.E. The Wind is a phenomenon of spring, the season of the Liver. It comes and goes quickly, moves swiftly, and blows intermittently. It causes signs and symptoms to arise and change rapidly. Cold is the climate of winter, the season of the Kidney; it contracts and causes pain. Heat and Fire represent the heat of summer, the season of the Heart. Heat is an External Excess; Fire is an Internal Excess that usually converts from chronic Internal Heat. Dampness represents long summer, the center, the season of the Spleen. It is environmentally associated with high humidity and wet or damp places. Although Dampness is essentially seasonal in nature, living or working in a wet environment or wearing wet clothing can invite invasion by Damp pathogens. Summer Heat is the purely seasonal pathogen of the transition from long summer to autumn. It combines pure Heat and humidity symptoms. Dryness is the pathogen of autumn, the season of the Lung. Pestilential Qi, first posited during the Ming dynasty (1368–1644 C.E.), is identical to the Western concept of infectious disease caused by microbial invasion.

Externally contracted illnesses are generated when either the invading pathogen is too strong for bodily immunity to deal with effectively, or when the Correct Qi is so depleted that even minimally virulent pathogens are capable of establishing themselves within the system. The basic treatment strategy differs according to the underlying cause.

Attack: When illness is caused by the virulence of the invading pathogen, the primary focus of treatment is the elimination of that pathogen through the use of medicinal herbs that target the specific pathogen, either directly (e.g., by use of antibiotics) or by stimulating a bodily response to directly oust it (e.g., by use of purgatives or diaphoretics).

Supplementation: When mild or moderate pathogenic influences are allowed to establish a foothold because of a deficiency of Correct Qi, the primary approach to treatment lies first in boosting immune function through supplementation of the underlying deficiencies, and attacking the pathogen only after vital function is restored to normal competence. Oriental bodywork plays a vital role in this phase of treatment.

Internal Causes

Diseases arising internally are always manifestations of a preexisting imbalance between Yin and Yang. While externally caused diseases may arise from a Yin-Yang imbalance, creating inequality between a pathogen and the Correct Qi, the dysfunction is almost always one of Excess of either Yin or Yang and usually presents as an acute condition. Internally generated diseases, on the other hand, usually manifest as chronic Organ problems and can often be traced to a long-standing deficiency of Yin or Yang function. Here the therapeutic focus is placed on strengthening and nourishing the balance of Yin or Yang. If Blood is deficient it is nourished; if Qi is deficient it is boosted. Ultimately, of course, all dysfunction can be traced to an imbalance between Yin and Yang, and the focus on the struggle between the pathogen and the Correct Qi, or Yin and Yang, may shift during any illness. Accurate and timely evaluation of conditions is always the key to effective treatment.

Emotional factors play a major role in internal disease, both as causes and as manifestations. Chinese philosophical thought never reached the Cartesian separation between body, mind, and spirit that characterizes, and hampers, our medical culture. Our physical body, feelings, thoughts, and spirit form a continuum of manifestation, delineating the human being at all of its levels of interaction with Heaven and Earth.

Each of the Element/Organ complexes is in a reciprocal relationship with specific emotional states. Excessive emotions cause imbalanced functioning of the internal Organs, and inappropriate Organ function predisposes a person to specific, exaggerated, emotional affect. According to the *Nei Jing,* the seven emotions are Anger, Joy, Worry, Preoccupation, Sadness, Fear, and Shock.[3] These categories should not be interpreted too narrowly. The emotions affect the organs principally through their effect on Qi, and different emotions affect Qi differently. For example, Anger makes Qi rise excessively and affects the Liver. Joy slows the Qi, affecting the Heart.[4] Worry and Preoccupation knot the Qi, affecting the Spleen and Lung. Sadness dissolves Qi, harming the Lung. Fear makes Qi descend, affecting the Kidney, and Shock scatters Qi, affecting the Kidney and Heart. Most of the emotions, when intensely prolonged or repressed, cause Qi to stagnate, turning Heat into Fire.

Ted Kaptchuk points out that cultural factors, such as extreme overcrowding; a desire to save face;

the Oriental philosophical unity of the body/mind; and lack of a discrete, personal psychology, tend to cause Orientals to somatize emotional conditions, leading them to be presented and treated as somatic dysfunctions.[5] Whereas the Western emphasis on personal individuation focuses on bringing mental and emotional considerations into conscious awareness, allowing for mental/emotional integration and self-fulfillment, Oriental self-development is situation-centered, tending toward self-definition in terms of social context rather than individual personal development. Excessive cultural emphasis on equanimity and saving face render any expression of emotional affect as inappropriate. This extreme difference in social mores has generated a good deal of confusion in the transmission of Oriental medical culture to the West. The emphasis our culture places on expressing ourselves, analyzing, talking about our deepest problems, and delving into the past or into the darkest recesses of our minds is bewildering to the Oriental psyche and antithetical to the Oriental approach to feelings.[6]

Independent Causes

In addition to the internal and external pathogens we have already discussed, the Chinese recognize several other causes of pathogenesis: diet, excessive sexual activity, overwork, trauma, and parasites.

Diet

Health depends on the intake of a balanced mixture of the Five Flavors (sour, bitter, sweet, spicy, and salty). Excessive indulgence in any one flavor either indicates a preexisting Organ/Element imbalance or will create one. For example, constant eating of sour foods either indicates a Liver imbalance or will create one over time. Considerations about the timing of meals, as well as the cleanliness, quantity, and toxicity of the foods eaten, complete this category.

EXCESSIVE SEXUAL ACTIVITY

Compulsive sexual activity depletes Jing, harming the Kidney. Too frequent childbirth will also weaken the Kidney, as well as the Conception and Penetrating Vessels, affecting menstruation.

OVERWORK

Excessive indulgence in any one form of activity may prove harmful to the internal Organs and the general state of health. The *Su Wen* states: "Prolonged vision damages the Blood; prolonged lying damages the Qi; prolonged sitting damages the flesh; prolonged standing damages the bones; prolonged walking damages the sinews. These are the five forms of Overwork."[7] The Spleen is the Organ most vulnerable to overwork.

TRAUMA

Trauma medicine is a highly developed art in China. The Chinese people's long experience with the martial arts, and the close association between those arts and medicine, allowed them to develop very evolved strategies for immediate first aid in cases involving trauma. Traumatic injuries include impact trauma, incised wounds, burns and scalds, and poisonous bites. Bruising and fractures, common occurrences in a martial setting, caused schools of martial arts to evolve very precise hand-healing and herbal remedies for these conditions. Liniments for treating bruises and contusions, called "hit wines," are common to every martial arts tradition. Today in China the treatment of fractures is performed by bodywork therapists, and includes soft-casting and daily manipulation.[8]

PARASITES

Knowledge of parasitic invasion was extant from the Sui dynasty (610 C.E.) in China and was attributed to eating or drinking unclean food or water. Therapy for this condition is exclusively herbal.

Miscellaneous Factors

PHLEGM

Chinese medicine considers phlegm to be the viscid mucus secreted by the respiratory, digestive, and urinary systems. The Spleen is considered to be the basis of phlegm formation, although it may manifest in many other places, for example the Lung, Heart, or even the pathways. In all cases, phlegm congests and inhibits the functions of whatever body part it is located in.

STATIC BLOOD

Any impairment of the smooth flow of the blood within the circulatory system gives rise to Static Blood. This applies whether the blood is static within the circulatory vessels or has extravasated. Since this condition always impairs normal function, it is considered pathogenic.

WRONG TREATMENT

The final cause of disease is wrong treatment applied by the practitioner. Whereas the side effects of allopathic medicine are notorious, Chinese medicine, especially herbal medicine, can also exacerbate disharmony. For this reason, accurate pattern assessment is the prerequisite for appropriate treatment. This is true in bodywork, where an inaccurate assessment of the client's condition can lead to the use of techniques that only make the situation worse.

THE FOUR EXAMINATIONS

Because the Oriental physician of ancient times was limited to information that could be elicited through the senses, Oriental diagnosis developed in a hierarchy of levels, from subtle to gross. Beginning with the observations you make utilizing all of your senses as the client enters your office, and concluding with a hands-on examination on the table, the Four Examinations are called Looking, Listening and Smelling, Questioning, and Palpating. The purpose of this process is to aid in identifying the pattern of imbalance that has caused the client to come to see you. Primarily you will be examining the signs (information that you observe) and symptoms (information your client notices) in order to get a clear picture of the presenting condition. Appropriate treatment depends on accurate assessment. The signs and symptoms of Chinese medicine are much broader than those of Western medicine and are decidedly less "disease" oriented. They include all of the holographic sets of correspondences that have developed over the last two millennia. Thus, facial color can be a key factor in Oriental assessment, while it would be ignored in Western medicine. It is important not to jump to conclusions on the basis of only one sign or symptom. An accurate assessment requires a synthesis of all of the information provided by the Four Examinations.

Looking Examination

The first of the four diagnostic forms is called the Looking Examination. By observing such qualities as spirit, posture, movement, color, and facial lines, a master can discern 90 percent of the story before the patient says a word. While in training with my teacher, I would sit in the corner of his office and watch him scribble furiously in Japanese as each patient would enter the room, take off his or her coat, and sit down. My teacher would then turn the sheet of paper face down and proceed with the more tangible aspects of his evaluation. After finishing the treatment, he would show me what he had written before the first word was spoken. As a rule, he had already figured out 90 percent of the story.[9]

Looking offers the initial opportunity to assess your client. The person's spirit and physical appearance—including constitution, structure, bearing, and complexion—are the general arenas available to visual observation. Much data concerning internal organ function and the acute or chronic nature of the person's condition can be obtained in this manner. Assessment of the tongue, a major form of evaluation, is also considered under this category.

SPIRIT

Spirit refers to the vital quality of the client. Facial expression, complexion, posture, tone of voice, manner of speech, and the general tonus of consciousness are the qualities observed. It is said: "If the patient is spirited, he is fundamentally healthy; if he is spiritless, he is doomed."[10] Observations regarding the spirit of a client may be classified as spiritedness, spiritlessness, and false-spiritedness.

PHYSICAL APPEARANCE

Here the constitution, structure, bearing, and complexion of the physical body is observed. The constitution may be divided into Yin and Yang classifications. A robust and vital body with good color is considered Yang. A Yin body is thin, pallid, and dry, with low vitality. Structure consists of the symmetry of proportion, the usage of the various parts of the body, handedness, and disuse due to chronic patterns of pain. Bearing refers to the general comportment a client presents with, whether loud and active or quiet and passive. The complexion of the face reflects the condition of the entire system. The *Ling Shu* states: "The Qi and Blood of the twelve primary meridians and the 365 pathways rise to the face."[11]

The analysis of facial color is done in terms of the color correspondences of Five Element theory. Thus, black or dark brown indicates the Kidney, red indicates the Heart, white points to the Lung, blue-green indicates the Liver, and yellow-orange the Spleen. The *Nei Jing* presents two different schemata for facial diagnosis, one in the *Su Wen* and

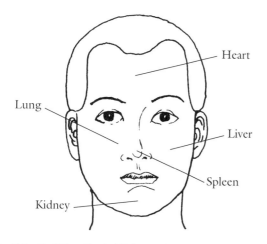

Fig. 5.1. Su Wen *Facial Diagnosis*

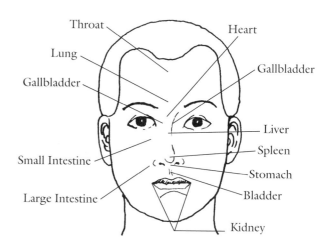

Fig. 5.2. Ling Shu *Facial Diagnosis*

the other in the *Ling Shu*. The *Ling Shu* distinctions are much more intricate, involving the Yang Organs. Lines, creases, and blemishes in these areas are also of diagnostic value. Figures 5.1 and 5.2 show these two schemata.

TONGUE DIAGNOSIS

Aside from these observations, the primary method of the Looking Examination is tongue diagnosis. Evaluating the balance of health and disease by observation of the tongue is a major pillar of traditional Chinese diagnosis. This method is based on a comparative analysis of the vitality, shape, color, and bearing of the tongue body, and the color, nature, and distribution of the tongue "fur," or covering. Tongue diagnosis has, since the second millennium B.C.E, been a definitive method of ascertaining the location and severity of pathogenic factors and determining the condition and prognosis of the body's recuperative powers.

Tongue diagnosis enjoys wide appeal for many reasons. Firstly, because the human system is so complex, recent events or very complicated conditions can present contradictory information at the time of your assessment of a client. Strong emotional experiences or recent physical exertion can easily give rise to contradictory signs in the pulse.

Because the condition of the tongue is relatively unaffected by short-term events, it is the most accurate indicator of the patient's true state. Secondly, the tongue is the most accurate indicator of the resolution or exacerbation of pathological conditions. The tongue body most clearly reflects chronic conditions, while the coating reflects acute changes. The third reason for the wide acceptance of tongue diagnosis as a definitive method for assessment is that there is broad consensus among various schools about the location of the various reflex areas of the tongue (fig. 5.3). As well, the information reflected on the tongue is relatively objective. A red tongue is a red tongue. Subtleties are always open to differing interpretations, but basic evaluation is a fairly straightforward process

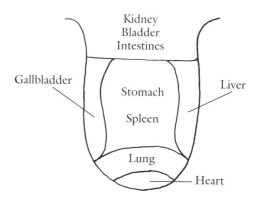

Fig. 5.3. *Tongue Correspondences*

in tongue diagnosis. Finally, tongue diagnosis is easy to teach and learn. Classroom instruction and clinical practice are both effective ways of training students in this approach.

The major drawback in using tongue diagnosis is its relative imprecision in locating finer pathological details. Pulse diagnosis, or the palpation of specific acupoints or meridians, is much more specific. This limitation merely warns us away from an exclusive dependence on tongue evaluation, which is completely in harmony with the traditional adjuration to always employ each of the Four Examinations in the evaluation process.

The protocol for tongue examination is very straightforward; it should always be done in the same fashion. Several conditions and considerations need to be kept in mind. Natural sunlight is the only way to get an absolutely correct reading of the tongue. Evaluation should always be done near a window, if possible. If this is impossible, incandescent light is better than fluorescent light, and strong light is better than weak. If only fluorescent lighting is available, the full-spectrum type is best.

The tongue should be completely extended, but without excessive force. This is important because overly forceful extension distorts both the shape and the color of the tongue. If prolonged extension is necessary for a clear evaluation, then repeated brief extensions of 15 to 20 seconds each will not adversely affect the process. The client should close his or her mouth briefly between extensions.

The appearance of the "normal" tongue conforms to the following characteristics. Body color should be a fresh, pale red color, like fresh meat. Considered an off-shoot of the Heart, and nourished by the "steaming" action of the Stomach, a pale red tongue body indicates an adequate supply of Heart blood and Stomach Fluids. The shape should be regular and without deformity or invol-

untary motion. The normal coating is thin and white, slightly thicker at the root than at the tip. Normal digestive function constantly sends a small amount of turbid dampness to coat the tongue surface. Moderate moisture is also normal; hence, the tongue should be neither too dry nor too wet.

Listening and Smelling Examination

LISTENING

The Chinese use the same word, *wen*, to denote both listening and smelling. The Listening Examination focuses on voice, respiration, and the manner in which a client talks about his or her condition. The location and quality of pain can be inferred from the way a person talks. Since joint pain is exacerbated by movement, people experiencing it attempt to remain as still as possible while speaking. Thoracic and diaphragmatic pain constrict the vocal apparatus, which leads to distorted vocalization. Cranial pain is exacerbated by the vibrations of speaking, and this leads to a very quiet, yet clearly enunciated, speaking voice. The Heart is the storehouse of the Shen, the consciousness, and energetic disorders of this Organ reflect in incoherent verbal responses.

The Five Element correspondences of sound and speech are also useful indicators of Organ/Element imbalances. These include a shouting voice for a Liver imbalance, a laughing voice for the Heart, a singing voice for the Spleen, a whimpering voice for the Lung, and a groaning voice for Kidney disharmony. These sounds can give you useful clues for further exploration.

SMELLING

Each Element/Organ complex produces a characteristic odor when pathologically afflicted. When the Liver is afflicted there is a rancid smell, Heart imbalance produces a burnt smell, Spleen dysfunction smells sweet, Lung pathology smells rank, and a diseased Kidney smells putrid. Halitosis is generally caused by Stomach Heat, although it can also be produced by stagnant food in the stomach or intestines, or by indigestion. Inflammation of the mouth, gums, teeth, or throat can also produce halitosis. Belching of sour, foul-smelling gas is due to damage to the digestive tract caused by excessive quantities, or poor qualities, of the foods eaten.

The Smelling Examination is best carried out discreetly during the palpation examination. Halitosis, or the severe olfactory cues of terminal cancer or advanced kidney disease, however, may well announce themselves earlier. Normal body odor, even from lack of adequate hygiene, is not relevant to this discussion, although in very extreme cases I have refused to treat clients until they have bathed.

Questioning Examination

Questioning the nature, cause, severity, and location of a client's problems is a primary tool in evaluation and treatment design. The *Su Wen* states: "If, in conducting the examination, the physician neither inquires as to how and when the condition arose, nor asks about the nature of the patient's complaint, about dietary irregularities, excesses of sleeping and waking, and poisoning, but instead proceeds straightway to take the pulse, he will not succeed in identifying the disease."[12]

At the time of the late Ming dynasty (seventeenth century C.E.), inquiry was considered to be "the essential element of examination, and the most indispensable of all aspects of clinical practice."[13] However, questioning always involves the risk of subjective considerations and can cause confused communication. This lack of absolute reliability in client communication merely points to the need to always employ each of the Four Examinations. Assessment should always be based on the total pattern of signs and symptoms that are presented.

The Ming dynasty physician Zhang Jie-Bin suggested the following protocol for the questioning examination:

1. Cold and Heat
2. Perspiration
3. Head and Body
4. Stool and Micturition
5. Diet
6. Chest
7. Hearing
8. Thirst
9. Identify Yin and Yang from the pulse and the complexion
10. Note any strong odors and abnormalities of the spirit

Later physicians modified this protocol to include medical history and environmentally related questions. These considerations include questions concerning the location and possible causes of pain and discomfort, the onset of the present condition, the specific time of the greatest discomfort, the predominance of Hot or Cold symptoms, patient preferences among the Five Element correspondences, previous medical (or structural) problems and related treatments, and working conditions.

Since BodyWork Shiatsu is a form of massage, you will receive a preponderance of complaints relating to soft-tissue injuries in clinical practice. Although the underlying cause of many somatic injuries lies in the Organ and energetic systems, it is necessary for Western practitioners to be able to screen injuries or specific areas of pain in anatomical terms. This will facilitate your communication with both your patient and other health professionals.

A final word about the Questioning Examination. People can frequently give you the most astute and accurate information about their condition. Asking with a sincere desire to hear what your client needs to tell you will often be the deciding factor in inspiring a high degree of trust.

Palpation Examination

Great exactitude and refinement of understanding is called for in this last, but by no means least, method of diagnosis. In spite of being the fourth phase of your evaluation, this is the most important part. The body is free of ego or falsehood and tells an exact and accurate story of its internal functions to the skillful palpation of the Oriental practitioner. Now you confirm the clinical impressions you have begun to formulate, based on the information you have gathered by Looking, Listening and Smelling, and Asking.

Our bodies are covered with a series of holographic diagnostic maps, each of which can tell the expert practitioner everything that is happening inside the human body. I witnessed an old Chinese doctor tell a friend of mine what her father died from simply by diagnosing her pulses! There are many reflex systems of diagnosis in use throughout Oriental medicine. Each method of examination forms a complete system of diagnosis and takes much practice to master. Included among these systems are diagnosis of the eyes, both the iris and the sclera, which reflect the entire body, as do the ears (with eighty-four acupoints each); the tongue; the hands and feet; the face; the front of the body; the umbilicus; and the back of the body. The tonus of the meridian and tendino-muscular pathway systems also allow the skilled practitioner to diagnose what is happening within the body.

PULSES

Traditionally, the palpatory technique most widely used by acupuncturists and herbalists is pulse diagnosis. Pulse-taking is among the oldest and most broadly practiced forms of medical diagnosis in the world. Every culture that has developed a literate medical system has independently developed this art.[14] By the time of the *Nei Jing*, in the early Han dynasty (100 B.C.E.), Chinese medical theory posited that Qi and Blood flowed together through the Blood Vessels (Jing Mai). Chinese physicians used pulse palpation at different locations around the body as a means of judging the relative state of both Qi and Blood, as well as the Organs, in the Three Heaters. A series of nine arterial acupoints reflecting the different Heaters was first used in this evaluation. These points, as described in the *Su Wen*, are located on the head, hands, and legs.[15]

The practice of using the radial styloid pulse was not established until the later Han dynasty (200 C.E.), when the *Nan Jing* (Classic of difficult questions) was published. The *Nan Jing* divided the radial pulse into three positions and three depths—the so-called "nine regions"—and related them to the Three Heaters. It said: "There are three positions, Inch (Cun), Barrier (Guan), and Foot (Chi), and three depths, superficial, middle, and deep. The upper position corresponds to Heaven and reflects diseases from the chest to the head; the middle position corresponds to the Person and reflects diseases between the diaphragm and umbilicus; the lower position corresponds to Earth and reflects diseases from below the umbilicus to the feet."[16] These correspondences are shown in table 5.1.

TABLE 5.1
Pulse Positions of the Three Heaters

POSITION	HEATER	AREA OF BODY
Inch	Upper Heater	Diaphragm to crown
Barrier	Middle Heater	Navel to diaphragm
Foot	Lower Heater	Navel to feet

The superficial level of the pulse is assessed by just resting the fingertips on the artery. The deep position is evaluated by pressing until the pulse stops, then backing slightly off. The middle position is felt in between these two positions. The three depths at which the pulse is taken have been assigned a variety of diagnostic interpretations over the years. The superficial pulse reflects the state of the Qi, exterior diseases, or problems at the surface of the body, as well as the health of the Yang Organs and meridians. The middle position reflects the state of the Blood, as well as digestive problems. The deep level reflects the general state of Yin, interior diseases or structural problems, and the Yin Organs and meridians. The left wrist reflects the left, or Yang, side of the body, while the right wrist reflects the right, or Yin, side.

Over the past two thousand years much consideration has been given to the different pulse positions and the Organs or meridians they reflect. The two best known, and still most widely used descriptions, come from the *Mai Jing* (Pulse classic), written in 280 C.E by Wang Shu He, which presents the meridian relationships from the point of view of acupuncture, and the *Bin Hu Mai Xue* (Pulse study of Bin-hu Lake), written in 1564 by Li Shi Zhen, who presented the pulse positions of the Organs as they were attributed to the Three Heaters in herbal medicine. From ancient times the Zang (Yin) Organs were considered to reflect at the pulse at positions analogous to their location within the Three Heaters. All schools of thought placed the Heart and Lung in the Upper Heater, with their pulses at the inch position, the Liver and Spleen in the Middle Heater, with pulses at the barrier positions, and the Kidney in the Lower Heater, with pulses at the foot positions.

Major disagreement came over the placement of the Fu (Yang) Organs and the nature of the Kidney. Different schools of Chinese medicine describe very different functions for the kidneys. The left kidney is assigned the same fluid-cleaning and urine-producing functions as are given in Western physiology. The right kidney, however, is considered the storage container for the ancestral Essence (Jing) we inherit from our parents and also assists the Heart in housing the Shen, or consciousness. Called Ming Men (Gate of Vitality), the right kidney is considered the "root" of all of the Yin and Yang Organs and the fundamental source of vital energy in the body. Some schools placed the kidneys at both foot positions; some assigned the right position to Ming Men.

The disagreement over the pulse positions of the Yang Organs has created confusion up to the present time. The pulses reflect both Organs and meridians. From the point of view of acupuncture, as detailed in the *Mai Jing*, the relationship between the meridians is preeminent, and the Yang Organs are linked to their Element-related Yin Organs. This places the Large and Small Intestines at the inch position in the Upper Heater, along with their Interior/Exterior-related Organs, the Lung and the Heart. The herbal point of view, espoused in the *Bin Hu Mai Xue*, gives priority to the Organs and places the Intestines by Heater location at the foot position.[17]

Modern Japanese acupuncture goes a step further and assigns the right foot position to the meridian functions of the Triple Heater and the Heart Envelope. This is based on the idea that the Source Qi is brought from Ming Men to the Source points of the meridians by the Triple Heater meridian and is thus the functional basis of Kidney Yang. The Triple Heater and Heart Envelope connect the Three Heaters, and most especially Ming Men, to the Heart. This focus on the meridian function of Source Qi distribution from Ming Men to the meridian Source points makes the representation of the Triple Heater and Heart Envelope much more useful in clinical acupuncture or bodywork practice than the Kidney/Ming Men differentiation of the herbalists.[18] Table 5.2 shows the correspondences between pulse position and Organs/meridians as currently used in Japan.

TABLE 5.2
Pulse Positions of the Organs/Meridians

POSITION	LEFT	RIGHT
Inch	Small Intestine/ Heart	Large Intestine/ Lung
Barrier	Gallbladder/ Liver	Stomach/ Spleen
Foot	Bladder/Kidney	Triple Heater/ Heart Envelope

Taking the Pulse

The pulse is taken by placing three fingers on the radial pulse. The barrier position is located on the radial artery level with the styloid process, the inch position is the finger space distal, and the foot position is the finger space proximal. The middle finger is placed at the barrier position, and the first and third fingers naturally fall on the inch and foot positions.[19] The finger spacing depends on the size of the patient: some space may be required between the fingers for taller people, while the fingers are closer together for shorter people. Infants require only one finger placed at the barrier position.

Traditionally, the pulses are taken in the early morning, before the Yang Qi rises for the day and while the Yin Organs are still calm. Needless to say, this is not practical in a professional practice. In any event, sufficient time should be given for the patient to quiet down and relax after arriving at your office. The patient should be sitting comfortably with wrists supported, or lying supine. The arm should be horizontal and no higher than the level of the heart. You must calm and balance your own breath before beginning to take the pulses in order to be able to accurately judge the rate of your client's pulse.

The pulse is first felt as a whole, using all three fingers. You must palpate each location for a minimum of five beats in order to get an accurate reading. Feel for spirit, root, and Stomach Qi. Feel the three levels to assess the Three Heaters, and also the surface, middle, and interior of the body. Compare the upper inch position with the lower foot position, and the left hand with the right hand, looking for balance. Last, feel the Organ/meridian positions, assessing the various qualities of the pulses.

The Normal Pulse

The normal pulse has three predominant qualities: having Stomach Qi, having spirit, and having root. The Stomach is the root of Post-Heaven Qi and the origin of Qi and Blood. Thus, it gives body to the pulse. A pulse with Stomach Qi is not rough. It is elastic, gentle, calm, and relatively slow—four beats per respiratory cycle. The *Su Wen* says: "The Stomach is the Root of the five Yin Organs; the Qi of the Yin Organs cannot reach the pulse by itself but it needs Stomach Qi . . . if the pulse is soft it indicates that it has Stomach Qi and the prognosis is good."[20] Spirit refers to the regular, steady qualities of the pulse. It should be soft but strong, neither big nor small, and steady in its qualities. Root refers to Kidney function. A pulse has root when the deep level can be felt clearly and also when the rear (foot) position can be felt clearly. A pulse with spirit, root, and Stomach Qi indicates harmony in consciousness, Qi, and Essence.

The Qualities of the Pulses

From earliest times various normal and pathological qualities have been assigned to each type of pulse. Over the millennia the number of qualities associated with the pulses has grown to twenty-eight. The first eighteen represent the primary disharmonies and can be grouped into seven categories: depth, speed, width, strength, shape, rhythm, and length. The other ten qualities represent variations of these primary qualities, and they present the extremely various and complex conditions found among the Organs and meridians. This picture is greatly complicated by the fact that pulses rarely manifest only one quality at a time. More commonly, they present as a composite of several distinct qualities simultaneously. Each position will present different qualities, according to the conditions of the Organ or meridian being assessed. These qualities are:

Depth: floating, sinking
Speed: slow, rapid, moderate
Width: thin, big
Strength: empty, full
Shape: slippery, choppy, wiry, tight
Rhythm: knotted, hasty, intermittent
Length: short, long

The other pulse qualities are flooding, minute, weak, soft, leather, hidden, firm, moving, hollow, and scattered.[21]

REFLEX-POINT EVALUATION

Several sets of acupoints are used by the Japanese for assessing the patient's condition. Japanese shiatsu primarily focuses palpation examination on point and area reflexes rather than pulse assessment. Tongue and pulse assessment are part of the Japanese anma tradition. Palpation evaluation is based equally on the objective tactile perception of hypertonic or hypotonic tissue at the acupoints and reflex areas, and the subjective quality of sensation in the patient elicited by palpation. Excess conditions manifest objectively in hot, tight, nodular tissue that resists pressure and subjectively elicits a sharp painful response in the patient. Deficient conditions objectively result in soft, boggy tissue that yields to pressure with an insubstantial, cold, or empty feeling to the practitioner and a discomfort that "hurts good" to the patient. Normal tissue, exhibiting balance, is essentially nonreactive. Tissue of normal tonus is springy, resilient, and vital and does not cause a notable sensation when compressed. We will review three sets of diagnostic points—Associate, Alarm, and Source points—and the most traditional abdominal reflex map.

Note: The acu-inch is a variable unit of measurement utilized in Oriental medicine. The acu-inch is based on the body proportions of the person you are treating. As a general measure, have the person bend the middle finger. The distance between the middle two lines on the side of the finger equals his or her acu-inch.

Associated Points

Shu (in Chinese, or Yu in Japanese) points reflect the sympathetic nervous system balance of the Organs and meridians on the dorsal surface of the body.[22] *Shu* means "associated" or "advertisement" and is an indication of the way in which these points reflect an imbalance in the functional energy associated with each Organ. Meridian problems first manifest in the Associated points. These points are located paravertebrally, 1½ acu-inches lateral to the dorsal midline (third sagittal standard line), between the levels of adjacent spinous processes (fig. 5.4). Starting with the Lung Shu point, Bl 13, the Shu points lie in the middle of the erector spinae muscle group, on either side of the spine. (Exceptions are the two most caudal Shu points, which are at the level of the first and second sacral foramina, overlying the lateral edge of the sacrum.) The closer the reactive point is to the spine, the more acute the reflected imbalance. Although traditionally located directly on the Bladder 1 meridian, chronic problems will frequently be found at the designated level but more lateral on the Bladder 2 meridian, and imbalances just beginning to occur can be palpated next to the spinous process in the lamina groove. This groove is not considered a traditional meridian but rather a series of related points. The Japanese call it Seki Sai Sen, which means "next to the spine." The Chinese refer to these points as Hou Tuo's Jia Ji points.

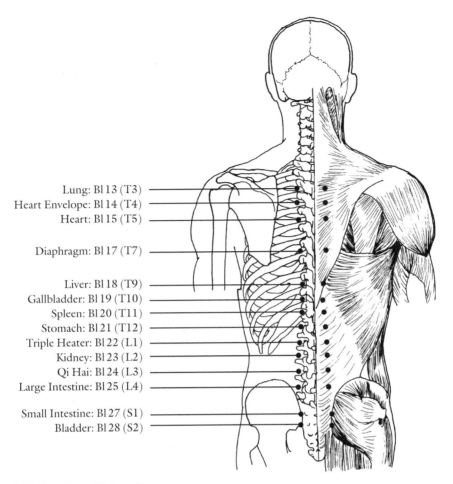

Lung: Bl 13 (T3)
Heart Envelope: Bl 14 (T4)
Heart: Bl 15 (T5)

Diaphragm: Bl 17 (T7)

Liver: Bl 18 (T9)
Gallbladder: Bl 19 (T10)
Spleen: Bl 20 (T11)
Stomach: Bl 21 (T12)
Triple Heater: Bl 22 (L1)
Kidney: Bl 23 (L2)
Qi Hai: Bl 24 (L3)
Large Intestine: Bl 25 (L4)

Small Intestine: Bl 27 (S1)
Bladder: Bl 28 (S2)

Fig. 5.4. Shu (Yu) Associated Point Chart

The active Associated points may frequently be seen as swollen or hollow areas depending on their Excess or Deficient condition. Temperature and color differences from the surrounding tissue are obvious. Although points reflecting Excess conditions are always more obvious, care must be used to palpate equally for the less obvious Deficient conditions. Just as meridian problems can be unilateral, so can Shu point reflexes. They tend to be most prominent on the same side of the body as their physical organ. These are effective treatment points and are frequently used for organ problems. Skin defects found on Shu points usually indicate an inherent weakness in the related organ. Pimples or sores indicate that detoxification of the organ is either in progress or called for.

Alarm Points

Mu (in Chinese, or Bo in Japanese) means "alarm" or "warning." The Mu points reflect the more Yin, parasympathetic nervous system, Organ functions on the ventral surface of the body (fig. 5.5).[23] As energetic imbalances begin to adversely affect the internal organs physically, these points become reactive. These reflex points are small, and care needs to be used in finding the exact location. Once the point is located, palpate gently to feel for textural or temperature changes on the skin. Then, exert pressure slowly, from superficial to deep, in order to see whether a response is elicited from your client. The more gently and superficially you are pressing when you get a response from your client, the more serious the imbalance. Responses elicited only on deep pressure indicate a less chronic, more easily correctable, condition of imbalance.

The locations of the Alarm points are as follows:

Lung (Lu1). One acu-inch below the inferior edge of the clavicle at the infraclavicular fossa, between the second and third ribs. To locate this point, have your client laterally abduct the arm to a 90-degree angle and raise it up a few inches from the table. The fossa will be obvious.

Heart Envelope (CV17). On the center line of the sternum (first sagittal standard line), where the nipple line (second transverse standard line) crosses it, between the fourth and fifth ribs.

Liver (Li14). On the mamillary line (third standard sagittal line) in the space between the sixth and seventh ribs.

Heart (CV14). One acu-inch below the tip of the xiphoid process, on the linea alba (third transverse standard line).

Gallbladder (Gb24). Slightly lateral to the mamillary line (third standard sagittal line) at the inferior margin of the seventh rib, where the cartilage of the eighth rib attaches to the seventh.

Stomach (CV12). Midway between the Heart Mu point (CV14) and the umbilicus, on the linea alba. This point normally lies on the middle arcuate tendon of the rectus abdominis.

Large Intestine (St25). One and one-half acu-inches lateral to the umbilicus, in the middle of the rectus abdominis muscles (bilateral). This point is normally found in the umbilical arcuate tendon of the rectus abdominis.

Qi Hai (Sea of Qi) (CV6). One and one-half acu-inches below the umbilicus, on the linea alba. This point is normally found at the inferior margin of the greater omentum. Qi Hai Mu is the anterior reflex point for the energetic center of the body.

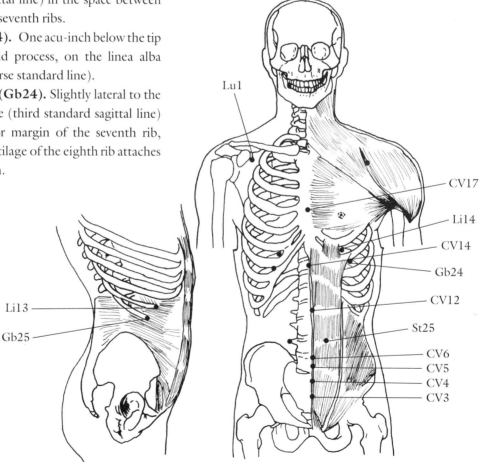

Fig. 5.5. Alarm Point Chart

Triple Heater (CV5). Three acu-inches above the pubic symphysis, on the linea alba.

Small Intestine (CV4). Two acu-inches above the pubic symphysis, on the linea alba.

Bladder (CV3). One acu-inch above the pubic symphysis, on the linea alba.

Spleen (Li13). Immediately distal to the tips of the eleventh ribs.

Kidney (Gb25). Immediately distal to the tips of the twelfth ribs.

Although the Alarm points tend to reflect the Organs and the Associated points tend to reflect the meridians, a response in only one set of these points does not constitute a definitive diagnosis of an Organ problem. Energetic imbalances and meridian disturbances ordinarily occur before Organs are affected; hence, they are reflected first and are much easier to resolve. When both sets of points are reactive, and so are the Source points, the situation is more serious. Please be careful in your communications with your client regarding the "meaning" of reactive points. Because we use the same words for the physical organs in the English language as we do for the functional Oriental Organ systems, it is easy to create misunderstanding and fear in a client's mind by casual remarks. Be mindful.

Source Points

The Yuan (Yo in Japanese) Source points near the wrists and ankles are used to confirm imbalances related to either Organs or meridians (fig. 5.6).[24] These points are where the central energy of the body is brought to each meridian by the Triple Heater, and they become reactive in either Organ or meridian problems. They are specifically used for the treatment of Organ problems. They are very helpful in confirming Shu or Mu point reactions and also in differentiating Shu or Mu point diagnosis, when the exact point that is reactive is uncertain. This can happen when the Shu or Mu points are in close proximity and excess adipose tissue prevents a clear assessment.

The locations of the Source points are as follows:

Lung (Lu9). At the transverse wrist crease, between the tendons of the flexor carpi radialis and abductor pollicis longus.

Heart (Ht7). At the ulnar margin of the transverse crease of the wrist radial to the flexor carpi ulnaris tendon, between the ulna and the pisiform bone of the wrist.

Heart Envelope (HE7). Between the tendons of the palmaris longus and the flexor carpi radialis, at the transverse wrist crease, in the flexor pollicis, on the tendon of the flexor digitorum profundus.

Large Intestine (LI4). Between the first and second metacarpal bones, through the first dorsal interosseous muscle, over the transverse head of the adductor pollicis.

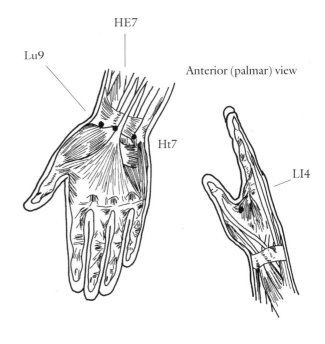

Fig. 5.6 Source Points

Triple Heater (TH4). On the dorsal wrist crease, between the carpal bones and the ulna, between the tendons of the extensor digitorum and the extensor digiti minimi.

Small Intestine (SI4). At the skin color change line of the ulnar aspect of the hand, proximal to the fifth metacarpal, in the depression distal to the pisiform bone, lateral to the origin of the abductor digiti minimi.

Spleen (Sp4). Along the skin color change line of the foot, distal and inferior to the base of the first metatarsal bone.

Kidney (Ki3). Even with the high point of the medial malleolus, midway between the malleolus and the Achilles tendon.

Bladder (Bl64). On the skin color change line on the infero-lateral edge of the tuberosity of the fifth metatarsal, on the inferior margin of the abductor digiti minimi.

Gallbladder (Gb40). Antero-inferior to the tip of the lateral malleolus, between the

malleolus and the talus, in the depression lateral to the tendon of the extensor digitorum longus, on the origin of the extensor digitorum brevis.

Liver (Li3). In the hollow between the bodies of the first and second metatarsal bones, in the interosseous muscle lateral to the tendon of the extensor hallucis longus.

Stomach (St42). At the high point of the dorsum of the foot, in the depression between the second and third metatarsal bones and the cuneiform bone.

Ling Shu Abdominal Reflexes

The Ling Shu reflexes were first described in the *Nei Jing* and are sections of the abdomen that become reactive when the Yin Organs are dysfunctional (fig. 5.7). They can manifest as sensitive, swollen areas from the surface of the skin down to

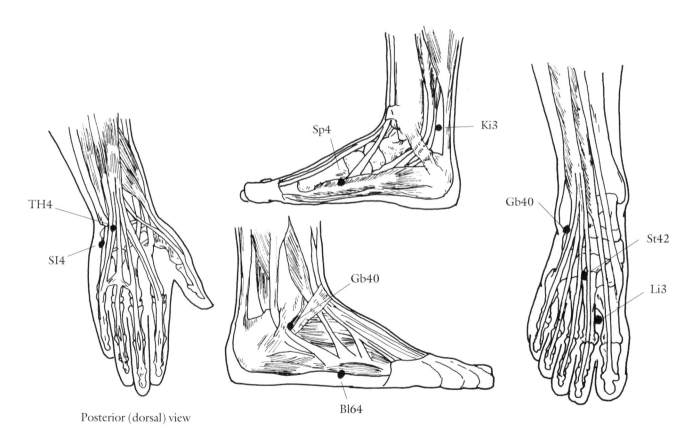

Posterior (dorsal) view

Fig. 5.6   Source Points (continued)

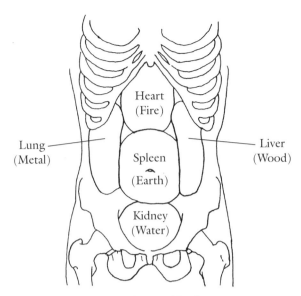

Fig. 5.7. Ling Shu Abdominal Reflexes

the core of the abdomen, depending on the severity of imbalance reflected. The ancient Chinese considered only the Yin viscera as critical, hence this simplified pattern. It is based on Daoist cosmological correspondences of directions in the body. Many modern practitioners have developed much more detailed maps.[25] Once the patient is on the table, these four sets of points are the major reflexes I use to refine and confirm my evaluation. I also use them to confirm local palpatory findings made during treatment.

CATEGORIES OF PATTERN IDENTIFICATION

Western medicine and traditional Chinese medicine differ radically in the methods used to evaluate disease conditions and design treatments for them. Western medicine focuses on the disease itself, treating disease states as independent entities that need to be diagnosed and named before treatment can be applied. Once the disease is identified, treatment protocol is determined on the basis of a preset approach to conquering the particular disease being treated regardless of the specific presenting conditions of the patient. This approach can often result in cures that are worse than the diseases that necessitate them. We are also left with a host of conditions that fall through the diagnostic cracks in the system, subclinical imbalances that produce no discernible organic degeneration yet result in a tragic diminution of the quality of life. One of the results of this approach is our present "disease-care" system with its enormous costs and the concomitant total lack of understanding of the realities of preventive health care.

Chinese medicine, on the other hand, developed an approach to treatment based on the evaluation of the total condition of the person at the time of treatment. This includes an evaluation of a person's history, living and working environments, diet, and mental and emotional conditions, as well as an assessment of the total pattern of presenting signs and symptoms. Treatment design using this approach does not require a specific disease "entity" to target for therapy but aims instead at the re-creation of homeostatic balance. This allows the bodymind, in effect, to cure itself. When this approach is utilized, each treatment becomes a unique event based entirely on the pattern of relationships formed by the constellation of signs and symptoms presented at the time of treatment.

Pattern identification reflects the naturalist Chinese tendency to emphasize relationship over structure. Specific signs or symptoms do not have a fixed meaning and can be interpreted only in terms of their relationship to all of the other signs and symptoms being presented. The enormous complexity of the human system, with the almost unlimited range of imbalances it is capable of manifesting, makes some system of classification for presenting signs and symptoms a critical prerequisite to treatment design. Successful treatment design depends on accurate assessment. Pattern identification allows for discernment of the nature, character, and location of the presenting condition and the creation of an appropriate treatment strategy. Chinese medicine has developed many such filters over the millennia.

Traditional Chinese medicine is a complete medical paradigm addressing all of the conditions that afflict humanity. Thus, some of the following filtering patterns are used mainly by herbalists, whereas others are focused on the needs of physical medicine. Internal medicine is primarily the province of herbology in Chinese medicine. Acupuncture, moxibustion, and bodywork are secondary to the use of herbs in treating internal organ diseases but play a more primary role in structural and orthopedic disorders. While early TCM focused primarily on acupuncture, this trend has gradually shifted, and now herbal medicine is preeminent in China. The different focus of these two branches of TCM has resulted in different forms of pattern identification. Additionally, the Chinese medical sciences had to deal with different kinds of pathologies at various times in their history, such as environmentally caused illnesses or epidemics of contagious febrile diseases.

These different focuses have produced several different ways of organizing information about the patterns of imbalance. The various kinds of pattern identification generally in use are all based on the Eight Principles. Subsidiary filters include those of the Qi, Blood, and Fluids; the Internal Organs; Pathogenic Factors; the Six Stages; the Four Levels; the Five Elements; the Three Heaters; and the Meridians. These filters are not mutually exclusive but are usually used in conjunction with one another to allow the physician to refine assessment clearly enough to enable effective treatment.

Not all of these methods of gathering information are useful in the practice of BodyWork Shiatsu. The primary arena for Oriental bodywork treatments involve the exterior of the body. The points and pathways, along with the neuromuscoloskeletal system, are our primary targets. Although we can help with the treatment of neurological, circulatory, endocrine, digestive, eliminatory, and reproductive problems, in general bodywork is only an adjunct modality in the treatment of internal organ diseases.

For the sake of a thorough review of TCM, I will briefly describe all of these identification patterns. Because of its importance, I will present the Eight Principles in some detail. The Oriental bodywork community *primarily* treats problems of the exterior of the body, skin, myofascia, and meridians, and the most relevant and familiar patterns are those of the Five Elements and the meridians. I will present the meridian identification patterns in greatest detail at the end of this section. For a more thorough treatment of these topics, see *Foundations of Chinese Medicine* by Giovanni Maciocia and *The Web That Has No Weaver* by Ted Kaptchuk.

Eight Principles

All Chinese philosophy, including medical theory and practice, derives from the fundamental discrimination of phenomena into the dialectical classifications of Yin and Yang. Over the course of time, Chinese physicians found that other distinctions were necessary to enable them to thoroughly describe all of the different imbalances that occur within the human bodymind. Beginning with the authors of the *Nei Jing*, many complementary pairs of opposites, in addition to Yin and Yang, have been used at different times to describe the clinical landscape. These have included Blood and Qi, Pathogenic and Defensive Qi, acute and chronic, falling and rising, damp and dry, thin and thick, soft and hard, lower and upper, Mucus and Fire, and still and moving, as well as the three pairs now used: Interior and Exterior, Cold and Hot, and Excess and Deficient. At the beginning of the Qing dynasty (late seventeenth century C.E.), the four pairs of opposites now in use were first named the Eight Principles (Ba Gang) by Cheng Zhong Ling in his book *Essential Comprehension of Medical Studies*.

Yin and Yang

This is the primary polar differentiation the Chinese use to categorize all of the phenomena of the universe. Yin and Yang may then be further differentiated into six subdivisions that cover all possible disease conditions. These are Interior or Exterior, Excess or Deficient, and Hot or Cold. The Interior, Deficient, and Cold parameters are all Yin patterns of imbalance, whereas Exterior, Excess, and Hot are all Yang patterns. According to this framework, the concrete manifestations of disease can be categorized within the abstract concepts of Yin and Yang. The Eight Principles allow all of the signs and symptoms observed during the Four Examinations to be woven into a basic description of the nature and location of every possible pattern of disease. While this description alone is sometimes sufficient to enable the practitioner to design an appropriate treatment, in general the Eight Principles give only a broad outline, which requires further refinement in order to yield specific treatment guidelines. Thus, for example, a classification of an Interior pattern of disharmony requires further refinement as to the specific Substance(s) affected, as well as the particular Organ(s) involved, before the correct treatment can be prescribed.

Interior and Exterior

This category differentiates the surface of the body from the inside. The Exterior consists of the skin and muscles as well as the pathways. The Interior refers to the organs and bones. Within the Eight Principles, Interior and Exterior refer to the location and characteristics of the signs and symptoms of disease

rather than to their causes. This is in contradistinction to the causes of disease, wherein the external (or Exterior) causes refer to the patterns created when environmental influences react with Correct Qi, mimicking the meteorological influences for which they are named, while the internal (or Interior) causes point to the effects excessive emotions have on the Yin and Yang functions of the body.

It is impossible to be specific about the signs and symptoms of Interior or Exterior diseases without further differentiating the effects of Cold and Heat and Deficiency and Excess, but in general, Exterior patterns involve the skin, muscles, and pathways and are acute in onset. Interior patterns are more chronic, involving the Organs and Substances.

Excess and Deficient

Excess (or full) conditions usually result from the conflict between an invading external pathogen and the Defensive Qi, or an obstruction of some sort causing a pathological buildup of Blood or Qi in the tissues or pathways. Deficient conditions indicate insufficient Qi, Blood, or Fluids, or underactivity of the Yin or Yang aspects of any of the Organs.

Hot and Cold

Cold patterns can arise from internal or external causes. Internal cold is generated when there is not enough Yang Qi to heat the body. External cold occurs when the body is unable to expel a cold pathogen. Both of these causes require a Deficient predisposition. Heat patterns can develop from external heat, deficient Yin fluids, or excessive Yang.

In clinical practice these simple patterns are rarely, if ever, seen. Usually, patterns are complex combinations of these parameters. Several Yin or Yang factors may combine to produce reinforced patterns, or Yin and Yang factors may present simultaneously to produce modified patterns.

Over time, parameters may convert from one polarity to another, and opposing polarities may manifest simultaneously in different parts of the body.

It is common for Excess and Heat, both Yang parameters, to be present together. Such a pure Yang pattern occurs when the Yin of the body, represented by the body fluids, is normal, but the Yang, in the form of heat, is in excess. This is usually caused by external factors. In such a case the presenting pattern is a combination of the patterns of the two parameters.

Deficient Cold is a pure Yin pattern. This is a Deficient pattern produced by chronic internal imbalance. Yin is normal but Yang is Deficient, making Yin appear relatively Excess; hence, this pattern is also called Deficient Yang.

When parameters of both Yin and Yang combine, as when there is Deficient Heat, the presenting pattern is a modification of the two factors. This pattern, called Empty Fire, is due to an insufficiency of Yin fluids causing normal Yang to appear in relative Excess, and is also known as Deficient Yin. Another mixed Yin and Yang pattern is Excess Cold. Here the pattern is caused by an excess of Yin (cold) while the Yang is normal. Although usually of external origin, this condition may arise from an internal deficiency. Here too the pattern is a mixture of the two parameters. This pattern is called Excess Yin.

Pure patterns, such as two Yin factors like Deficient Cold or two Yang factors like Excess Heat, are relatively simple to treat. Excess patterns must be reduced, while Deficient patterns need to be supplemented. Treatment is more complex in mixed patterns, as the more powerful influence is not always apparent. Pattern dominance may be determined by such factors as the time of day when symptoms manifest. Thus, the subtle hyperactive signs of Deficient Yin, which would not be apparent during the activity of the day, become obvious as insomnia at night, while the hypoactive reflection of Deficient Yang is more obvious during the day, when a more active state is normal. In this fashion, the relative predominance of Yin or Yang may be determined.

FALSE SIGNS

At the end range of both Yin and Yang disease patterns, contradictory signs, called Illusionary Cold or Illusionary Heat, can appear. These are extremely critical signs that Yin or Yang is coming to the end of its capacity to exert the normal restraints on the body's functions. Thus, a terminal Yang Heat disorder may suddenly present cold limbs. This sign is called True Heat/Illusionary Cold because the Cold sign is due to the extreme Yang forcing the remaining Yin to the extremities. The complementary situation, when there is a last flicker of Apparent Heat in a terminally Yin condition, is called True Cold/Illusionary Heat. This occurs when the Yang becomes so deficient that it floats to the surface before extinguishing.

COMBINATIONS:
CONVERSIONS AND COMPLEXES

Combination patterns are very common. These can occur when a person with a preexisting condition, for example Internal Deficient Cold, is attacked by an external pathogen that superimposes its pattern on the first. The precise signs in combination patterns depend on the relative strength of the different disharmonies. Another very common occurrence is for one pattern to change into another. With every change in condition the appropriate treatment changes; this is why an evaluation is done at every session. Complexes present another possibility. These conditions occur when a new imbalance attacks before all the signs of the old one are eliminated or when a pathogen affects the exterior and interior simultaneously. Complexes can also occur when one part of the body is affected by one pathogen while another part is attacked by a different pathogen entirely.

As you can see, the Eight Principles offer a broad and inclusive framework within which we can gain a general understanding of the myriad signs and symptoms of human disease. Accurate diagnosis, however, usually requires further refinement by other assessment patterns, especially those of Qi, Blood, and Fluids, and the Organs, to allow for pinpoint accuracy in treatment.

Qi, Blood, and Fluid Patterns

Qi, Blood, and Fluid patterns are used to further refine Eight Principle pattern evaluations regarding possible pathological changes to the Essential Substances. This filter is used in conjunction with the Organ patterns to further locate the exact site and nature of dysfunctions causing the presenting Eight Principle pattern. There is some overlap between these patterns and the basic Eight Principle patterns. Qi dysfunctions can be characterized as Deficiency of Qi, Sinking of Qi, Stagnation of Qi, and Rebellious Qi. Blood patterns are Deficiency of blood, Stasis of Blood, Heat in the Blood, and Loss of Blood. Fluid patterns include Deficiency of body Fluids, edema, and phlegm.

Organ Patterns

Organ patterns are the most clinically useful differentiations in chronic internal organ diseases. The Organ pattern filter is essentially an application of the Eight Principles to the Qi and Blood imbalances of the Organs. It is used to further refine diagnosis in order to indicate the specific Organ or Organs underlying the symptoms being presented. An Eight Principle diagnosis of Qi Deficiency, for example, is not clinically useful in treatment design until the involved Organ, usually the Lung or Spleen, is indicated. This allows for specific treatment to be applied.

The real art of Oriental diagnosis lies in being able to discern the underlying patterns with the least available number of signs and symptoms. Organ diseases present on a gradient, from newly forming conditions with symptoms just emerging to chronically entrenched diseases with all symptoms fully present. The earlier in this progression the pattern can be assessed, even while relatively few signs or symptoms are present, the better the chances of obtaining a lasting cure. The best physician needs the fewest clues.

With very few exceptions, Organ patterns do not duplicate Western diseases. They are an expression of the underlying disharmonies that generate the signs and symptoms observed in the Four Examinations and are therefore extremely useful in determining the treatment necessary to resolve the presenting complaints. In practice these patterns can occur singly, but frequently they are present in many combinations. Combinations can include two or more patterns from one Organ, patterns from two or more Organs, patterns from both Yin and Yang Organs, and Organ/meridian complexes.

Pathogen Patterns

When we reviewed the causes of disease we looked at the meteorological factors of Wind, Cold, Summer Heat, Dampness, Dryness, and Heat (Fire) as external pathogenic causes of disease. When used for the diagnosis of disease, these patterns, external or internal, mimic the effects of external pathogen invasion in the body. They present as the pattern of the meteorological condition within the body, whether the actual pathogen is present or not. You need not have been exposed to external Cold, for example, in order to manifest Cold signs and symptoms. In clinical practice, what is important is the pattern of a pathogenic factor, not the presence of the actual climactic condition. Pathogens can reflect as either internal or external patterns, depending on their cause. In general, external genesis presents with an acute onset, and internal genesis presents more gradually.

Six Stages, Four Levels, and Three Heaters

These three categories of pattern evaluation are concerned with the diagnosis and treatment of serious infectious and epidemic diseases, principally through the use of herbs. Because of the symptom-related focus of Chinese medicine, pattern identification can differentiate the depth, or the energetic layer or level, to which a pathogen has penetrated the body, thus determining the appropriate herbal treatment. These three filters focus on the body from several distinct but related points of view, allowing the physician to choose the appropriate category of herbs to use for each stage of these internal disease processes.

SIX STAGES

Two thousand years ago, in the time before antibiotics and the general awareness of the need for personal and community hygiene, epidemics of typhoid fever and other environmentally borne cold diseases were the major killers of the population. Up to 70 percent of the deaths were caused by Cold-induced diseases, resulting from external pathogenic invasion.[26] Shortly after the time of the writing of the *Nei Jing*, at the end of the later Han dynasty (200 C.E.), one of the greatest Chinese physicians of all time, Zhang Zhong-Jing, evaluated diseases caused by external Cold in a book called the *Shang-han Lun* (Discussion of Cold-induced disorders).

Zhang evaluated the disease process initiated by invasion of external Cold, which enters the body and then converts into a sequence of other internal patterns. He classified six stages of intensification of the disease process, corresponding to the sequential progression of the meridian pairs of the Six Energies. These are Tai Yang (Bladder and Small Intestine); Yang Ming (Stomach and Large Intestine); Shou Yang (Gallbladder and Triple Heater); Tai Yin (Lung and Spleen); Shou Yin (Heart and Kidney); and Jue Yin (Liver and Heart Envelope). Only the Tai Yang stage reflects an external (Cold) condition. The other stages represent all of the various converted internal conditions of febrile disease.

As we saw in the section on the Eight Principles, the Excess or Deficiency of a disease is determined by the balance between the strength of the pathogen and the strength of the Correct Qi. Excess occurs when both the pathogen and the Correct Qi are strong, and the conflict between the two produces Excess symptoms. Deficiency occurs when the Correct Qi becomes unequal to the task of repelling the invader, and the pathogen succeeds in penetrating the interior of the body.

Zhang's system also delineates the depth to which the pathogen has penetrated. In the three Yang stages the disease is still superficial, affecting the Yang meridians and Organs; the pathogen is predominating over the Correct Qi, producing signs of Excess Heat, and treatment is targeted at eliminating the pathogen. The Yin stages represent a deeper penetration to the level of the Yin Organs; the pathogen, though still present, is weakened, as is the Correct Qi, and treatment focuses on strengthening the body's Qi.

FOUR LEVELS

A means of gauging the depth of penetration of external Heat diseases was developed during the early Qing dynasty, in the mid-eighteenth century, by Ye Tian-Shi in a book called the *Wen Re Lun* (Discussion of Warm-febrile diseases). At that time Warm-febrile diseases, infectious diseases caused by external Heat, were the major killers of the population.[27] Treatment for febrile diseases caused by external Cold had earlier been dealt with in the Six Stage differentiation of the *Shang-han Lun*.

On the basis of clues from both the *Nei Jing* and the *Shang-han Lun*, Ye developed a system of classifying the symptoms of Heat penetration based on the Yang-to-Yin gradient from Qi to Blood. Qi is the underlying foundation for all manifestation and exists on many different levels of density, ranging from the most rarefied energies to the densest fluids. Ye distinguished four progressive layers of pathogen penetration: the Wei (Defensive Qi), the Qi, the Ying (Nutrient Qi), and the Xue (Blood). Wei and Qi represent the Yang portions of the body in this spectrum, while Ying and Xue reflect the Yin aspects. Energetically they range from the most superficial level of Yang to the deepest layer of Yin in the body. Although designed to describe the advancing stages of external Heat, the Four Levels equally describe the pattern of internally generated Heat diseases of the Ying and Xue.

THREE HEATERS

Infectious febrile diseases caused by external Heat, such as measles, scarlet fever, and smallpox, continued to be the major killers into the nineteenth century, when Wu Ju-Tong systemized and extended the work of Ye and others in the *Wen Bing Tiao Bian* (A systematic differentiation of febrile diseases). Wu presented the concept of depth in the body from the vertical perspective of the Three Heaters. In this schema the Upper Heater is the most external part, the Middle Heater more interior, and the Lower Heater the most interior. The Three Heater schema is used to assess the vertical penetration of external Heat in conjunction with the Four Level assessment of the energetic depth and severity of the disease.

Five Element Patterns

Although the Five Element patterns can be used to diagnose conditions that we recognize as diseases, their greatest value lies in recognizing the signs and symptoms of imbalance as soon as they manifest, long before disease develops. The previously discussed patterns are all relevant only for a condition that has already established itself. Unlike the other filters, the Five Element patterns have been developed more for their predictive value in preventive health care than for the diagnosis of patterns of disease.

Over millennia of observation, practitioners noted the numerous correspondences to the functional health or imbalance of each Organ system. By observing such minutiae as the quality of a person's fingernails or his or her preferences in foods, the general balance of all of the internal systems could be assessed. Treatment could then be directed at restoring complete, harmonious balance long before the disease pathogenesis recorded by the other pattern filters occurred.

Imbalances occurring within the Five Element paradigm take place in the Creation and Control cycles. Control Cycle problems manifest as the Overwhelm, and Rebellion cycles. Although the Organ patterns are much more clinically useful in diagnosing internal organ diseases, some energetic conditions fall through the cracks in the Organ patterns but are reflected by the Five Element patterns. Creation sequence patterns describe Organ deficiencies induced by the mother element on the Creation Cycle. Overwhelm sequence patterns are created when an Organ exerts inappropriate control over another Organ on the Control Cycle. In this sequence, note is made of facial color, as that is the indicator of the origin of the disharmony. The rest of the presenting symptoms usually derive from the imbalance created in the overcontrolled Organ. Rebellion sequence patterns occur when a severely Excess Organ rebels against the Organ that normally controls it, harming the controlling Organ.

Meridian Patterns

Meridian patterns are the oldest form of pattern recognition developed by Chinese medicine. The information from the *Han Ma-wang* (Burial mound silk books) shows that knowledge of the meridians even predates recognition of the acupoints themselves. Although these patterns are described in detail in the *Nei Jing*, the actual development of this knowledge predates that book by many centuries and lies rooted in the earliest recognition of the interplay of Yin and Yang, especially the relationship between the surface of the body and the inside.

Chinese medical practitioners recognized the unity of the Organ/meridian complex very early. They saw that Organ pathology always affects the meridians and is reflected in them, and that meridian pathologies also affect their respective Organs. They also noticed differences between Organ and meridian pathologies. Meridian problems present as distinct patterns and can occur without concomitant Organ problems. Pathology of the meridians frequently precedes Organ involvement, as meridian imbalance represents the energetic end of the energy↔matter continuum. It is necessary to distinguish these patterns in order to chose appropriate treatment.

Meridian pathology can be initiated in four ways. Firstly, environmental pathogenic factors can invade the meridians directly, causing pain, numbness, Heat, or Cold according to the nature of the pathogen. These pathogens can also settle in the joints, causing Painful Obstruction Syndrome, or further invade their respective organs. Secondly, overuse of a limb or body part, in sports or work, can cause Qi stagnation in the related meridians.

Thirdly, orthopedic injuries can cause Qi stagnation or can injure the meridians directly. Finally, internal organ imbalances eventually cause injury to their related pathways.

Aside from the sets of related signs and symptoms that have been accumulated by observation over the millennia, meridian pattern identification must include an assessment of the relative Excess or Deficiency of the affected pathway. When Excess conditions are present, meridians feel hard, swollen, and stiff to your touch and feel contracted and sore to your patient. Pressure elicits sharp pain. Excess Heat or Cold are apparent visually as a red or blue coloration to the pathway, as well as by a palpable variation in temperature. Deficient conditions present as flaccid and depressed meridians that feel cold, look pale, and respond to pressure with a dull ache that "hurts good."

The *Nei Jing*, as well as most modern texts, give the signs and symptoms of meridian pathology mixed together with those of the related Organ pathology. Because the Organ patterns are a much more refined and effective filter for identifying Organ dysfunction than the meridian patterns, I will give only the symptoms of the primary meridians and the tendino-muscle pathways in this section. Note that some of the traditional symptoms given for the Yin meridians are actually symptoms of the related Yang meridians. For a more in-depth review of the traditional signs and symptoms of all the pathways, see *Acupuncture: A Comprehensive Text* by O'Connor and Bensky.

LUNG

Primary pathway: Fever; aversion to cold; stuffiness of the chest; pain in the clavicle, shoulders, and arms. *Tendino-muscle pathway:* Stiff, strained, or twisted muscles and pain along the course of the pathway; muscle spasms over the upper anterior ribs; bloody sputum.

LARGE INTESTINE

Primary pathway: Sore throat, toothache, bloody nose, runny nose, swollen and painful gums, swollen eyes, pain along the course of the meridian. *Tendino-muscle pathway:* Stiff or strained muscles along the course of the pathway, inability to raise the arm at the shoulder, inability to move the neck from side to side.

STOMACH

Primary pathway: Pain in the eyes, bloody nose, swelling of the anterior neck, facial paralysis, cold legs and feet, pain along the course of the meridian. *Tendino-muscle pathway:* Strained muscles of the third toe, muscle spasm in the front of the lower leg or thigh, spasm in the foot muscles, swelling in the front of the pelvis, hernia, spasm of the rectus abdominis, spasm of the anterior neck or cheek, wry mouth, muscle spasms of the eyelids that prevent either opening or closing of the eyes, Bell's palsy.

SPLEEN

Primary pathway: Vaginal discharge, cold feeling along the meridian, weakness of the leg muscles. *Tendino-muscle pathway:* Strain of the muscles of the big toe; sprain or pain in the medial muscles or joints of the ankle, leg, thigh, or groin; strain in the upper portion of the rectus abdominis.

HEART

Primary pathway: Pain in the eyes, pain on the inner side of the arm, pain along the scapula. *Tendino-muscle pathway:* Cramping inside the chest, stiffness or strain of the muscles along the course of the pathway.

SMALL INTESTINE

Primary pathway: Pain in the lateral neck, pain in the elbow, stiff neck, pain along the lateral side of the arm and scapula. *Tendino-muscle pathway:* Stiffness or pain of the muscles of the pinky finger, pain or stiffness of the joints or muscles along the course of the pathway, strained levator scapula or scalene muscles, ringing earache, pain from ear to jaw, vision problems.

BLADDER

Primary pathway: Fever and aversion to cold, headache, stiff neck, pain in the lower back, pain in the eyes, pain behind the leg along the course of the meridian. *Tendino-muscle pathway:* Pain or spasm of the muscles or joints of the little toe, the heel, the calcaneal tendon, the calf, the posterior knee or thigh, the sacrum, the paravertebral muscles, the axillary region, the back of the neck or base of the skull; pain radiating superficially from the base of the skull to the forehead.

KIDNEY

Primary pathway: Pain in the lower back, pain in the sole of the foot. *Tendino-muscle pathway:* Muscle spasm or pain in the sole of the foot or along the muscles or joints of the postero-medial aspect of the ankle, lower leg, or thigh; stiffness of the spine on flexion or extension.

HEART ENVELOPE

Primary pathway: Stiff neck, pain along the course of the pathway, contraction of the elbow or hand. *Tendino-muscle pathway:* Pain or spasm along the course of the pathway, superficial chest pains.

TRIPLE HEATER

Primary pathway: Pain along the course of the meridian, pain in the elbow, alternating chills and fever, deafness, pain and discharge from the ear, pain at the top of the shoulders. *Tendino-muscle pathway:* Pain or spasm along the course of the pathway, a curled tongue.

GALLBLADDER

Primary pathway: Alternation of chills and fever, headache, deafness, pain in the hip and lateral side of the legs, pain and distension of the breasts. *Tendino-muscle pathway:* Pain in the fourth toe, painful rotation of the ankle at the lateral malleolus, pain along the peroneal muscles or at the lateral edge of the knee, pain or sprain of the tensor fasciae latae, pain in the hip joint extending to the groin or the deep buttocks, sacral pain radiating to the lower ribs, pain in hypochondriac region, lateral rib or neck pain, inability to move eyes from side to side.

LIVER

Primary pathway: Headache, pain and swelling of the eye, cramps in the legs. *Tendino-muscle pathway:* Strain of lateral muscles of big toe; pain on the front of the ankle; pain of the medial part of the knee joint; pain or spasm of the medial thigh muscles; pain, contraction, or flaccidity of the genitals.

PART 2

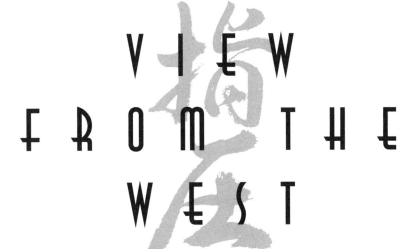

VIEW FROM THE WEST

CHAPTER 6

THE EFFECTS OF BODYWORK SHIATSU: A WESTERN PERSPECTIVE

WHAT FOLLOWS IS REASONED speculation based on equal parts of research, practice, analytical thought, and intuition. These theories attempt to explain the effectiveness of BodyWork Shiatsu in light of the latest Western scientific findings. In the following discussions we will proceed from the microscopic to the gross and systemic, from specific effects to broad theoretical considerations.

CELLULAR CHANGES

Cell Function

Normally, cells die when the buildup of internal toxic and/or metabolic wastes literally chokes them to death. I conjecture that increased intracellular pressure on the cell membranes forces very small and marginally lodged waste material through the cell wall pores, discharging this waste material in a way that is not otherwise possible. This produces a direct, rejuvenating effect at the cellular level, enhancing cell function and increasing cellular metabolism. Since the number of times that each cell can accurately reproduce itself is genetically determined at birth, the longer each cell functions effectively before it dies, the longer the associated tissue exists in a state of health.

Histological Effects

When soft tissues are strongly stimulated by digital compression, they release several pro-inflammatory enzymes, notably histamine, serotonin, brady-kinin, and prostaglandin(F).[1] These pro-inflammatory amino acids initiate a supercompensatory* immune system response. In those areas where deficient Qi energy flow is due to the buildup of metabolic or toxic residues, or where

*Supercompensatory or heterostatic changes reflect the extraordinary return to homeostasis of an overwhelmed biological system when challenged by a "heroic stimulus." This describes not only the effects of BodyWork Shiatsu but also the progressively enhanced stages of physical conditioning created by the incremental increases in training efforts by athletes.

postinfectious or post-traumatic cellular debris have been insufficiently removed, this inflammatory response is often enough to cause the body to clean up the debris and return normal tissue function and energy-flow characteristics.

Another histological effect that takes place in connective tissue occurs when these tissues are irritated by deep compression. The mast cells present release the enzyme hyaluronidase, which acts on a chemical level, in conjunction with the electrocolloidal processes described below, to loosen the molecular bonds of the ground substance. This facilitates the shift from gel state to sol state in matrix material (hyaluronic acid), making it possible for the manipulations of BodyWork Shiatsu to free up and rebalance myofascial structures.

MUSCULOSKELETAL SYSTEM

Digital compression, the major technique of BodyWork Shiatsu, works in three ways to lengthen (and consequently relax) muscles and tendons. The first two form the basis of neuromuscular massage, and the third, the basis for myofascial bodywork techniques.

Muscles

The medulla oblongata, the oldest and most basic part of our brain, contains an ongoing program that determines the resting length of every muscle fiber in the body. Controlled by feedback from the proprioceptive portion of the central nervous system, this muscle resting-length program allows the body to maintain the balanced flexor/extensor tonus necessary to keep us upright against the force of gravity. This program also contains the lifetime record of the insults and traumas of life.

Muscle length and tonus is monitored by neuromuscular fibers called muscle spindles. These lie parallel to the main muscle fibers, attaching to the muscle fibers or to their tendons. Appearing among the true myofibrils, muscle spindles are either chain fibers or bags of stretch-reactive nuclei, according to the type of muscle they are in. Each spindle is wrapped by several different specialized nerve fibers and has its own independent neurological connections. They are connected to their tendinous insertions by miniaturized myofibrils called intrafusal fibers. These intrafusal fibers are capable of contracting or relaxing independently of the extrafusal fibers of the main muscle mass, regulating their length. The intrafusal fibers act as the control mechanism for the feedback loop that allows the central nervous system to maintain the appropriate flexor/extensor tonus that keeps us continuously balanced in gravity.

The intrafusal fibers also act as an early warning system, providing feedback when the muscle/tendon complex is being stretched too fast or too far. Control for this mechanism acts through the internuncial neuron pool within the spinal cord. When activated by being stretched too quickly or beyond their preset limits, the muscle spindles initiate a neurological feedback reflex that causes the entire muscle they are part of to contract. This prevents the muscle fibers from being torn loose from their attachments. This is the effective mechanism of the "knee jerk" test doctors use to evaluate neurological function when they tap the patellar tendon with a rubber mallet.

Muscle spindles are also the culprits responsible for maintaining the joint imbalance related to myofascial strains long after the actual muscular or fascial trauma heals. This happens because the nervous system lacks an effective mechanism for resetting hyperfacilitated muscle spindles. Without appropriate manual intervention, strains can return whenever the affected tissues are stressed, as every athlete knows.

By mechanically lengthening muscle fibers through compression, and maintaining that stretch long enough for the proprioceptive feedback system to complete its feedback loop (usually three to five seconds, although it can take much longer in muscles contracted due to hyperfacilitated neural pathways or by imbalanced meridian Qi), the brain will reset the involved muscle resting-length pattern.

Tendons

The medulla also monitors tendons and the joints they cross over and move. This is done with a group of proprioceptors made up of Ruffini end-organs, Pacinian corpuscles, and Golgi tendon organs. The feedback from these mechanisms allows for unconscious awareness of the angulation of joints; the rate of, and resistance to, change in that angulation; and their position in space. They work in coordination with the muscle spindles to give us our extraordinary ability to be aware of and to control the incredible range of activities of which our muscle/tendon complexes are capable.

The Golgi tendon organs perform a complementary function with the muscle spindles in protecting the muscle/tendon complex from injury. They reflexively inhibit muscular tonus when they are suddenly stretched with too much force and simultaneously cause a stimulation of antagonist tonus, effectively inhibiting the activity that led to their overstimulation. This allows the body to accommodate stresses that otherwise might tear tendons free from their bony attachments. Having your leg buckle when you unexpectedly stumble on the stairs, thereby avoiding injury to the myofascial tissues of the leg, is an example of this mechanism.[2] The Golgi tendon organs are affected by compression in the same fashion as muscle spindles, making BodyWork Shiatsu effective in tendon-related injuries.

Skeletal Structure

In the Orient they do not make the distinctions we do between therapeutic massage and bodywork, physical therapy, and chiropractic treatment. A certified Oriental bodywork therapist is trained in the techniques necessary to maintain skeletal alignment.

Skeletal alignment is important for two major reasons. The first is that misaligned joints impede normal nerve function and nutrition by pinching the emerging nerve roots in the narrowed intervertebral foramina. These impingements cause pain at the site of the misalignment and interfere with the bodily functions mediated by the involved nerves by impeding neurological transmission. Nerve-root compressions lasting for extended periods of time can permanently damage not only the nerves themselves, but also the structure and function of the tissues they control. Modern chiropractic physicians have documented numerous muscular and organic dysfunctions correctable solely through realignment of the subluxated joints that cause the neurological irritation.[3]

The second major problem caused by misaligned joints is the effect they have on balance in the muscular system. Muscular imbalances affect structural integrity, causing circulatory and organ dysfunction by altering the spatial relationships necessary for the normal operation of these systems.[4] The abnormal muscular tension produced also adversely affects the vital energy flow through the meridian system. This creates localized excesses or deficiencies in the flow of Qi, which can also affect Organ function. These energetic imbalances are always part of the destructive feedback loop that leads to the improper function of the muscle groups involved.

In addition, a less critical but still important consequence of joint imbalance is the restriction in normal range of motion that is produced. Though not normally life-threatening, the problems caused by restriction of normal movement can range from merely inconvenient to incapacitatingly painful.

Because BodyWork Shiatsu addresses muscular tonus as well as Qi flow, restrictions in free joint movement relieved by this approach are much less traumatic to the tissues involved, and the realignments produced are of much longer duration, at times bringing permanent relief with only one treatment.

MYOFASCIAL SYSTEMS

In the living body all muscular fibers are encased within a webwork of fascia. Called the perimysium, this "skin" around the myofibrils is continuous with all of the other fascial coverings of the muscle and joins together at the ends of the myofibrils to form the tendinous insertions on the bones. Tendons insert by fusing with the periosteum, the skin that covers the bone. This is an important point. Although we talk about the various fascial components as if they were different entities, using different names for different functions or locations, the fascial system is one contiguous network from head to foot. Not only are all of the fascial components part of one inseparable whole, but they are functionally inseparable from their bony or muscular complements. Muscles, bones, and fascia form one integrated system. In the following discussion we will consider the fascial component by itself, remembering that this is only an intellectual distinction and not a separate system.

Fascia
Fascia is the most ubiquitous material in our bodies, comprising 70 percent of the nonaqueous material of which we are made. It is generically called connective tissue. Tendons, ligaments, cartilage, bones, periosteum (the skin around bones), perimysium (the skin around muscles), and fascia (the inner "skin" around everything) are some examples. These tissues all derive from the embryological mesoderm. As the name implies, connective tissue is the material that holds everything together.

All connective tissue is basically the same—matrix material made up primarily of hyaluronic acid, collagen fibers for stability, elastin fibers for those tissues that stretch, various mineral salts for those tissues that are weight-bearing, and various cellular components to maintain the life processes.

Hyaluronic acid, or ground substance, is a colloidal protein. That means that it can exist in two different states, depending on its energy content—just like water and ice. In the normal, low-energy condition, ground substance is in its gel form, with the molecules tightly bound together. But as the energy level rises, through the addition of heat, pressure, or electrical charge, the matrix material transforms to its sol state. The molecules loosen their bonds and connective tissue stretches out. This is what happens when you warm up before exercise and your body becomes looser and more flexible.

Digital compression acts through three mechanisms to transform hyaluronic acid from gel to sol. First, remembering high school physics, pressure equals heat. Thus, pressure acts to raise the temperature of the affected tissues and initiates a change of state in the local matrix material. Second, collagen is piezoelectric,* and the repetitive press and release technique of BodyWork Shiatsu generates minute, localized electrical charges that

---

* Piezoelectrical materials are semiconducting crystals that release an electrical discharge when they are deformed and released. See Robert Becker's *The Body Electric*.

also act to transform connective tissue to their sol state by raising the level of energy. The third mechanism is the release of the enzyme hyaluronidase by the mast cells when they are "irritated" by digital compression. Hyaluronidase is the enzyme that breaks the molecular hydrogen bonds that keep matrix material in its gel state. These three effects combine to produce local conditions wherein the matrix material transforms from gel to sol and the various collagen fibers may be lengthened or separated. This is the mechanism that allows manual intervention to free the body of the adhesions and contractures that are the cause of so much pain and restriction. This is the main physiological mechanism underlying connective tissue manipulations.

Fascial Electrodynamics

The body develops from three embryological layers: the ectoderm, the endoderm, and the mesoderm. From a structural point of view, the body may therefore be considered as a series of concentric tubes.

Ectodermic development creates the skin and nervous system. At the very center of the spinal cord is a hollow tube, the canalis centralis, that extends up into the brain as four ventricles and is surrounded by the various afferent and efferent tracts of the central nervous system. These are, in turn, encapsulated by the meninges (the pia mater, the arachnoid membrane, and the dura mater). The hollow spaces between layers of the meninges allow for the circulation of the cerebrospinal fluid, the nutrient medium for the central nervous system. The central nervous system in turn sprouts

the sensorimotor and autonomic nerve tracts. Finally, the skin, the body's external boundary, is also derived from the ectoderm.

In terms of digestion, the core of the body, derived from the endoderm, is a hollow tube from mouth to anus, supported by the internal organs. This core is surrounded by the neuromuscular and musculoskeletal systems.[5]

The spinal column, created from the mesoderm, is the mineralized connective tissue that provides protective support to the spinal cord. The spinal column is surrounded first by a fascial skin (the periosteum) that provides nutrient and structural support for the vertebrae. This core is covered by a layer of intrinsic muscles that enable subtle and refined movement, then by a second layer, the deep fascia, which connects, supports, and feeds the intrinsic musculature. These two layers are in turn contained within the extrinsic muscles that allow for larger, more powerful movements. The final sheath of the superficial fascia, continuous throughout the entire body, holds all the layers of the tissue together.

These membranes, differentiated during embryological development, are the phase boundaries that exist at the interface between different materials in living systems.* The phase boundaries are the place of generation and transmission of the electromagnetic fields that act to control the growth and stability of the system as a whole.

Between each of the successive tissue layers lies a flowing tide of nutrient fluids. In order for these fluids to flow freely between the layers of tissues that form the various sheaths of the body, as well as for these layers to slide easily upon one another, it

---

* The term *phase boundary* designates the region of contact between two dissimilar substances. The physical chemistry of solutions shows that the phase boundaries found whenever two or more different kinds of matter exist side by side generate electromagnetic force. There are innumerable such phase boundaries in any living system. Specific phase boundaries can be identified as the source of the voltage gradients that generate the fields being measured in living systems, even though their absolute magnitude is unknown. See H. S. Burr, *Blueprint for Immortality* (London: Neville Spearman Ltd., 1972).

is necessary for the fluids and their surrounding tissues to have appropriate ionic charges. An inappropriate ionic charge, either on the phase boundaries or in the fluids flowing between them, can result in electrostatic stickiness, leading to the clumping of the formed particles carried within these fluids (one cause, I suspect, of atherosclerosis). In addition, this stickiness may also cause adhesive contractures between tissues. Too great a buildup of intercellular fluid between layers of connective tissue not only cuts off individual cells from their source of nutrition, but also creates bipolar electrical imbalances that can lay the groundwork for the formation of imbalanced ionic charges along the phase boundaries.

Properly applied compression corrects intercellular fluid congestion; it also rebalances fascial electrodynamics by piezoelectrically releasing the appropriate electrostatic charges necessary to neutralize the ionic imbalance. This brings the incredibly complex interplay between nutrient fluid flow and internal biostructural feedback into balanced harmony.

This deep piezoelectrical stimulation also facilitates manual intervention in freeing up intrinsic myofascial adhesions. These adhesions often make refined and specific movement patterns difficult or impossible. Lack of intrinsic muscular freedom is often the root cause of structural deviations created by the repetitive and habitual use of the extrinsic musculature to compensate for intrinsic muscle incompetence. Chronic low-back pain related to hyperlordosis (swayback), as an example, is frequently caused by the overdeveloped quadriceps and shortened hamstrings that occur in compensation for an incompetent iliopsoas muscle (the intrinsic flexor of the femur).

Although these deep tissues are often not directly palpable, they can be freed of restriction and returned to normal range of motion and func-

tion by indirect manipulation. Releasing intrinsic restrictions results in freeing the larger extrinsic muscles of their need to compensate and brings relief of pain through the restoration of balanced structure and fluid flow.

SYSTEMIC EFFECTS

Fluid Dynamics

A large percentage of body mass is made up of the fluids that circulate within us, bringing oxygen and nutrients to the cells and removing metabolic wastes and toxins that are the by-products of the life process. These fluids are also the transportation system for both the humoral and cellular components of our immune system. Basically comprised of water, minerals, nutrients, various gases, large protein molecules that perform immune-system functions, and various cellular components, this fluid is essentially the same throughout the body, but is named for anatomical distinction according to location and specific content.

The fluid of the circulatory system is called plasma and contains hemoglobin molecules for gaseous metabolism, plus a variety of other formed particles that perform immune and maintenance functions. This fluid moves freely through the capillary walls, performing its nutrient-bearing and waste-removal functions for the tissues outside the circulatory system, and there it is called intercellular fluid. Fluid that enters into the body's sewer system for purification and return to the circulatory system is called lymphatic fluid.

Both the circulatory return system of deoxygenated blood (the venous system) and the sewer system of nutrient-depleted and waste-loaded fluid (the lymphatic system) are passive, muscle-operated pumping systems, as compared to the arterial blood supply that operates by the hydrostatic pressure of the beating heart and the elastically pulsing arteries.

In both venous and lymphatic systems, fluids are prevented from backing up by an ingenious system of one-way valves that only open in the direction of the heart. Compression, regardless of direction, always acts to facilitate this flow, since the fluids in these channels can only move in one direction. For this reason, compressive techniques are most effective in stimulating return circulation to the heart.

By stimulating fluid return toward the heart, compression also creates space in the lymphatic system for the body to dump excess intercellular fluids, mechanically expressing them into their return channels and recreating the space necessary for optimum cellular nutrition and the reestablishment of appropriate ionic balance throughout the system.

Cerebrospinal fluid (CSF) serves the same nutrient-bearing and waste-removal functions for the brain and spinal cord that intercellular fluid serves for the rest of the body. As the joints of the spinal axis, including the cranial sutures and iliosacral joints, become restricted in their complete range of motion, the dural sleeve surrounding the spinal cord, which serves as the vessel system for the cerebrospinal fluid, becomes constricted and impedes the free flow of CSF.

Restrictive lesions of the cranial, interspinal, or sacral joints can form for many reasons. Imbalanced Organ/meridian energies can cause uneven tonus in the paired intrinsic muscles that support and help create the appropriate span for each segment of the spinal axis, resulting in subluxed vertebrae. This creates a local torque in the dural sleeve that can ramify from one end to the other. Traumatic or chronic injuries or illness can do the same. Postural defects can also initiate this cycle.[6]

Any restriction in the CSF pumping mechanism—including the cranial bones, the choroid plexus, and ventricles of the brain, the iliosacral joints, and the dural sleeve—directly affects the function of the entire central nervous system by interfering with the delicate balance of micronutrients and electrolytes required for optimal neural function.[7] The gentle core mobilization of Body-Work Shiatsu creates movement at every section of the spinal axis, not only facilitating the movement of the CSF but encouraging increased production of CSF in the brain.

Organ and Glandular Functioning

Six of the eleven internal organs are directly palpable through the shiatsu/anma technique of ampuku. Two others are partially palpable and the remaining three can be indirectly manipulated through mobilization of the rib cage.[8] Over the course of time, through lack of exercise, improper breathing and diet, restrictive clothing, and accumulated stress (including the effects of electromagnetic pollution and normal aging), these organs build up increasing residues of sludge-like waste that interfere with their normal functioning. This occurs both because of toxic poisoning and because the cells are mechanically choked.

For the solid Yin viscera, as with all tissues, compression forces out stagnant or toxic materials, bringing a rebound hyperemic flush of fresh arterial blood in its wake and stimulating a return toward normal function through detoxification. The Yang organs are all hollow tubes with a surface structure comprised of smooth muscle tissue. As the tonus of these tissues is controlled in part by visceral autonomic reflexes that affect smooth muscle tonus the same way that the muscle spindle apparatus controls skeletal muscle tonus, compression and jostlation (see page 101) are effective in restoring relaxed and unrestricted movement to bowel structures, and hence a return to proper function.

In Oriental medicine the Organs are considered to control the functioning of the joints, tendons, ligaments, hair, skin, bones, and so forth. Because of the relationship between the Organs and their meridians, Organ health always results in increased strength and pliability of the muscles through which each meridian runs. By creating balanced function in the Organs, all other bodily functions also improve.

All of the internal organs and endocrine glands, whether directly palpable or not, are normalized in their function both by the reflexes of the somato-visceral acupoint system and by the electromembranous (see appendix 3) balancing effects of meridian treatment. Because of the profound effects shiatsu has on the health of the internal organs it is considered primary care by the Japanese Ministry of Health and Welfare.[9] Although no system of manipulation can claim to cure internal organs in a state of gross and advanced degeneration, dysfunctions based on imbalanced energy flow are frequently and dramatically improved, and the ongoing process of degeneration can often be slowed or stopped. This is also true for organs whose function has been compromised by restriction in their normal range of movement due to trauma, toxicity, or disease.

When the energy imbalance that is the root cause of organ dysfunction is corrected, the body's own intrinsic healing power can produce miraculous cures. Even for the individual in normal health, regular BodyWork Shiatsu almost always has the effect of improving organ and glandular function. Thus "normal" health, usually considered as the absence of disease symptoms, transforms into the radiantly vital condition of true balance.

Whole Body Energy

Beyond all of the various specific effects produced by BodyWork Shiatsu, there is an augmentation of the total bio-electromagnetic energy field that is the subtle manifestation of all the various electrical, neural, magnetic, and fluid systems interacting properly. BodyWork Shiatsu creates a buoyantly energetic sense of lightness, vitality, and freedom from pain that is the result of the appropriate interaction and unrestricted function of the innumerable energy fields and physical systems that make up a human body.

THE CYCLE OF IMBALANCE

Because the body represents such a complex, interwoven web of biochemical, electromagnetic, neuroendocrine, visceral organ, and structural/mechanical relationships, imbalance at any level tends to ramify throughout the entire system. The delicate balance of true health is vulnerable to upset in many ways. Stress, trauma, improper diet, invasive microorganisms, toxic materials, lack of exercise, restrictive clothing, and excess electromagnetic radiation are among the many factors that can initiate dysfunction among the body's many systems.

Once initiated, by whatever cause and in whichever system, a pernicious cycle of imbalance tends to form, perpetuating and extending the disease process. A steadily increasing challenge is presented to the body's inherent homeostatic and self-healing properties.

For example, an imbalance initiated at the level of organ dysfunction, whether caused by poor diet, toxic insult, stress, or the invasion of microorganisms, will affect the energetic flow through associated acupuncture points and pathways; as they begin to reflect the imbalanced state of the related organs, the points and pathways will carry or reflect an inappropriate energetic charge.

As organ dysfunction continues to deepen, the departure from energetic balance will cause the flow of Qi to deviate further and further from normal. This in turn will reflect in the myofascial tissues through which the pathways flow. As dysfunction continues to increase, these myofascial tissues will begin to reflect excessive or deficient Qi flow by becoming hyper- or hypotonic. This development can have far-reaching consequences, since myofascial tonus is responsible for creating and maintaining appropriate span in the skeletal system, as well as for maintaining the spatial relationships between the nerves of the neural plexii, which are necessary for the proper functioning of the nerve plexus itself.[10]

This is especially true at the Shu/Yu point reflexes in the paraspinal musculature. The erector spinae muscle group is responsible for both gross movement of the spinal column and the maintenance of good posture. As the Shu/Yu points begin to react to Organ-pathway dysfunction, they begin to create an asymmetrical tonus in the muscles wherein they lie. This produces an imbalance of the supporting muscles of the individual vertebral segments of the spinal column. This is why we can perform certain actions every day of our lives, and then suddenly, while reaching for a book or bending over to tie a shoe, a nerve pinches and we are frozen in pain. I speculate that Shu/Yu point imbalance is the mechanism responsible for most chronic subluxing of vertebral segments appearing from unknown causes. These spinal problems are not successfully treatable by traditional chiropractic adjustments—they recur almost immediately. Because they result from a muscular imbalance due to Organ dysfunction, the cause of their appearance is most often not apparent, and treatment plans comprised only of mechanical adjustments are therefore not effective.

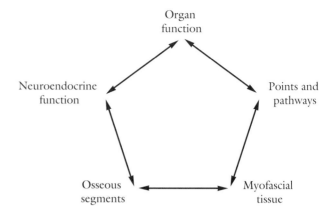

Fig. 6.1. Cycle of Imbalance

Subluxed vertebrae impinge upon the nerve roots entering or exiting the spine at the subluxed segment, creating agonizing pain and interfering with the organ and/or endocrine functions controlled by the affected nerves. This, in turn, deepens the organ dysfunction, and the cycle continues and deepens. This relationship may be visualized by the diagram in figure 6.1. Because the cycle is circular, it can be initiated by sufficient insult to any of its parts. The effects of imbalance cascade throughout the entire system, creating the chronic dysfunctions which we are resigned to accept as the normal consequences of life.

By intervening at any appropriate level of this cycle, BodyWork Shiatsu allows for the creation of what Dr. Hans Selye termed the heterostatic effect.[11] That is to say that when the body's own homeostatic capacities for returning the organism to balance are overwhelmed by the degree and complexity of dysfunction, the skillful intervention of a BodyWork Shiatsu therapist can initiate a supercompensatory response that enables the body to rebalance itself, setting the stage for the dynamic restoration of vital health.

In terms of preventive health care, evaluation made through the energetic system allows for breaking a cycle of imbalance long before the pathological degeneration of internal Organ systems reaches the degree of actual tissue necrosis by which allopathic medicine recognizes and diagnoses disease. Understanding the interrelationships between structure and function in the human system allows for remediation of the causes and symptoms of disease, and the noninvasive nature of Oriental therapies saves the patient from the often debilitating side effects of the cut and drug approach of modern allopathy.

STRUCTURE AND FUNCTION

I will here expand the commonly accepted definitions of *structure* and *function* to include an energetic viewpoint that clarifies the essential unity of these two concepts. We will examine structure and function first as they are understood in Western anatomical and physiological models, and then from an energetic perspective. We will finally consider how the various techniques of deep bodywork affect both structure and function.

Structure is defined by Webster as: "The way in which constituent parts are fitted or joined together, or arranged to give something its peculiar nature or character."[12] We normally think of the structure of a thing as its shape, as the framework that supports and creates that shape, and as the component parts of which it is made. We consider structure to be static and enduring. We tend to view the structure of something as an isolated event, discrete in time and separate from its function.

In defining *function* Webster is equally terse: "A characteristic activity or the activity for which something exists. The end or purpose."[13] *Taber's Cyclopedic Medical Dictionary* broadens this defin-

ition and develops it in a direction that begins to include the relationship between structure and function. Taber's defines *function* as:

The action performed by any structure. In a living organism this may pertain to a cell, or part of a cell, tissue, organ, or system of organs. The act of carrying on a specific activity. Normal function is the normal action of an organ. Abnormal activity, or the failure of an organ to perform its activity are the bases of disease or disease processes. Structural changes in an organ constitute pathological changes, and are common causes of malfunctioning, although an organ may act abnormally in the absence of observable structural changes.[14]

The relationship between structure and function now begins to become obvious, although we are still apparently dealing with a linear causal relationship rather than a reciprocal identity. Structure still appears to define function, and there is still a range of invisibility wherein the function of an organ "may act abnormally in the absence of observable structural changes."

When we view structure and function from an energetic perspective we realize the essential unity of these two concepts. We can see the full range of this relationship, from the proper function of appropriate structure to the complete dysfunction of degenerated structure. This includes all of those dysfunctional conditions that have not yet developed into discernable structural degeneration, where energetic imbalances have not yet begun to manifest symptomatically. Treatment at this stage, before symptoms begin to manifest, is the ideal of Chinese medicine.

From an energetic viewpoint, structure and function represent two poles of a single, multidimensional identity. In the Oriental paradigm, structure and function are complementary differentiations of the Dao. Structure equates with the earthy, solid, Yin pole, function with the heavenly, energetic Yang pole. Structure is the three-dimensional description of a static object in space. Function is the time-dependent, four-dimensional activity of that structure.[15] Any force that affects structure affects function, and any force that affects function affects structure equally and reciprocally.[16]

All deep-tissue bodywork techniques affect structure. The specific framework for evaluation and treatment design depends upon the levels of the organism addressed by the information base of the discipline. Whether addressing the microstructure of myofascial wound healing, as in sports massage, or fascial freedom and balance, as in Rolfing, or the sleeve/core energetic relationship, as in BodyWork Shiatsu, all deep-tissue techniques address human structure.

The structural changes induced by deep-tissue manipulation cause instantaneous change in the function of the affected tissues. At the neuromuscular level structure is influenced toward increased length, reduced muscle-fiber tension, separation and broadening of muscle fibers, freeing of adhered tissues, enhanced fluid circulation, and normalized neuromuscular hypertonus. In the myofascial tissues of the body these changes create increased strength and range of motion, decreased toxicity, reduced pain, greater metabolic function, faster rebound from use or trauma, and complete freedom of myofascial movement. All of these changes in function help to induce a parasympathetic rebound in the autonomic nervous system

that compensates for the sympathetic dominance found in chronic stress states, leading to the reestablishment of autonomic balance.

Structurally-oriented bodywork techniques address fascial balance and freedom. This affects all of the functions dependent on the stereotaxic relationships* of the various parts of the structure. For example, the appropriate functioning of the various neural plexii, whether voluntary or autonomic, depends on the proper physical relationships between the components of the structures that contain and support them. Because neurological function is dependent on spatial relationships, the nervous system requires the appropriate span† between various components of the neural plexus in order for the timely propagation of appropriate sequences in the signals generated to take place.[17] For this reason the postural imbalances focused upon by structurally-oriented bodywork techniques always have decreased neurological function as a symptomatic component.

As discussed in appendix 3, the biofields of the body direct the development of the meridians that carry their charges and are simultaneously affected by the functioning of those meridians. The Extraordinary Vessel system which oversees the autonomic nervous system also requires stereotaxic integrity for proper function. In order for the meridians to align with the force fields along which they evolve and whose charges they carry, the structures they exist within must maintain appropriate span between their various components.[18] Distorted structure will always produce a restriction in the free flow of Qi. The deranged neuro-

---

* *Stereotaxis* refers to the three-dimensional relationship of objects to each other, especially as they relate to the time-dependent functions of the nervous system. A feedback mechanism used by the nervous system to control function is the very refined timing requirements regarding when signals in the neural plexii reach their destinations. The continued initiation of proper neural sequencing depends on this timing.

† *Span* refers to the distance between two extremities. In the body, *span* refers to the relationship between structural elements that maintain balance in the myofascial system. This refers to the alignment of the bones in reciprocal relationship to the myofascial tissues that contain and support them.

logical function that always accompanies distorted structure is produced because the Yang, system-organizing information being carried by the various Yin structures is restricted in its flow.

In addition to the purely structural changes fostered by all deep-tissue techniques, BodyWork Shiatsu takes advantage of the point and pathway information system to directly alter function by tonifying or sedating the level and intensity of Qi flow. Altering the flow of Qi changes the tonus in the tendino-muscle channels, thus influencing myofascial span and leading to the return of more efficient functioning in the structures being treated. This direct effect on function, supported by the Oriental medical information base, helps to achieve energetic homeostasis by simultaneously addressing both structure and function.

STRESS

Stress can be loosely defined as the rate of wear and tear within the body. The human organism is designed to function optimally within relatively narrow limits, and constantly strives to recreate that homeostatic balance no matter how it is challenged. The constant interplay between the forces of change encountered in daily life and the homeostatic mechanisms of the body is one of the prime determinants of the quality and duration of life.

Within limits, the stresses of change are not only unavoidable but are necessary to the health and growth of the organism. A life without challenge lacks spice, and the very process of growth implies constant change. It is only when we are pressed beyond the limits of our ability to rebound into balance that stress becomes debilitating.

Dr. Hans Selye, the father of modern research on the effects of stress, defines stress as: "the state manifested by a specific syndrome which consists of all the non-specifically induced changes within a biologic system." He named this state the general adaptation syndrome (GAS).[19] Selye found that when stress is of sufficient intensity and duration, the organism undergoes an adaptive transformation that allows for an effective response to short-term stressors, but ultimately leads to systemic exhaustion and the onset of stress-related diseases that have replaced infectious diseases as the major cause of suffering and death in our culture.[20]

The GAS develops in three stages: alarm, resistance, and exhaustion. In the alarm phase the entire system mobilizes its forces to confront the stressor, whether that be your significant other yelling at you or a taxicab screeching to a halt inches in front of you. All of the neurological and endocrinological events of the "fight or flight" response are initiated. The alarm state is activated when the hypothalamus, a major component of the diencephalon or interbrain, reacts to a perceived threat, real or imagined. It is at this level of the brain that the autonomic nervous system (ANS) is regulated.

The ANS is itself divided into two distinct but complementary parts. The sympathetic nervous system (SNS) is responsible for preparing the organism for action. Although capable of initiating specific responses in the body, when activated in response to a threat it tends to turn on all the switches at once. This phenomenon is referred to as mass discharge, and initiates the fight or flight mechanism. The characteristics of this condition are dilated pupils (to let in more light and allow better vision); a tight throat; a tense neck and upper back, with the shoulders raised; increased musculoskeletal tonus; shallow respiration; accelerated heart and pulse rate; cool and perspiring hands; a locked diaphragm; a rigid pelvis, accompanied by numb genitals and a tight anus; contracted flexor muscles in the legs, with the extensor muscles inhibited; increased blood supply in the head and trunk, with a corresponding decrease of blood in the periphery and gastrointestinal tract; suspended peristalsis; cortex activity tending toward the faster beta rhythms; and facilitated conductance in the neural net and reduced threshold of stimulation at the myoneural junctions. By engaging the fight or flight mechanism, the body is ready for instant action.

The parasympathetic nervous system (PNS), by contrast, acts specifically within the organism to engender a state of deep relaxation, fostering digestion, self-repair, and creative or intuitive thought. Termed the vegetative response, the characteristics of PNS activity are flushed skin; softened and lengthened myofascial tissues; facilitated enzyme synthesis and peristalsis; contracted pupils; controlled elimination; inhibited afferent neural signals; heightened stimulation threshold at the synapses and myoneural junctions; and cortex activity tending toward alpha, or even slower, rhythms. When the PNS is dominant, the body-mind is turned inward and a state of deep relaxation is engendered.

Endocrinologically, the glands mediating immune function are inhibited by the mass discharge of the SNS. The first endocrine gland to respond to stress is the adrenal gland, which consists of two parts, an outer shell or cortex that produces the pro- and anti-inflammatory corticosteroids, and an inner core or medulla that makes adrenaline and noradrenaline.

Adrenaline, the fear hormone, is responsible for the feeling of the sudden flush of excitement we experience when confronted by danger. Adrenaline mobilizes glucose from the liver into the bloodstream to feed the muscles; increases carbohydrate metabolism; dilates the arterioles of the heart and skeletal muscles; accelerates heart rate; increases circulatory blood volume; increases oxygen consumption and the production of CO_2;

relaxes the smooth muscles of the gastrointestinal tract; constricts the sphincter muscles; and dilates the bronchial musculature. Shallow breathing and anal contraction are among the subjective components of this response. By contrast, noradrenaline constricts arterioles, raising blood pressure, and has much less effect on blood glucose. It is considered the anger hormone.

Increased adrenaline acts in a closed feedback loop within the system, activating the pituitary gland. The pituitary releases adrenocorticotropic hormone (ACTH) and thyrotropic hormone (TTH). ACTH acts on the adrenal cortex to stimulate the production and release of pro- or anti-inflammatory corticosteroids, depending on circumstances. TTH stimulates the thyroid to produce thyroxine. Thyroxine increases metabolic rate; brings on nervous perspiration; creates a shaky feeling; produces a rapid heartbeat; stimulates deep and rapid breathing; and leads to rapid exhaustion. Thyroxine and adrenaline potentiate each other, and while adrenaline is released as an immediate response to stress, thyroxine comes into play only when the stress continues for a prolonged period.

It is at this point in the GAS that the body switches from the alarm phase to the resistance phase, with the most effective system, in reference to the stressor involved, mediating the body's response. This defense continues until the specific system under stress becomes depleted, and the GAS transforms to the exhaustion phase.

The exhaustion phase initiates another episode of acute stress, and the system returns to the alarm phase, ultimately handing control to the next most capable line of defense. This cycle repeats over and over until all of our defenses are exhausted, and at this point, according to our genetic, nutritional, or environmentally produced weaknesses, we develop one of the stress-induced illnesses that have become endemic in our civilization. It is generally conceded by the medical profession that cardiovascular disease, cancer, arthritis, and respiratory ailments are all stress induced. It is also thought that the immunosuppressant effects of stress are causitive of allergic responses and vulnerability to infection, a relationship that has clear implications in the connection between the HIV virus and full-blown AIDS. The list of stress-related disorders will likely grow as the medical establishment conducts further research on the relationship between mind, emotions, and health.

For optimal function, the autonomic nervous system requires a balance between the sympathetic and parasympathetic nervous systems. As in all of nature, it is only in the balanced interplay of complementary functions that the Yin and Yang components of our constitution can achieve the harmony required for true health. The problem inherent in our physical nature is the fact that the neuroendocrine system is a creature of habit. If the sympathetic neural pathways are continuously facilitated, the body establishes a pattern of sympathetic dominance, maintaining itself in the hypertonic fight or flight mode even after the causitive stressors have been resolved. A vestige of a less cerebral time in our evolutionary development, the fight or flight mechanism was an essential protective device when there were ferocious predators behind every bush and the ability to flee from, or defend against, a threat to life was vital to continued existence in an eat-or-be-eaten world. Unfortunately, the visceral reactions appropriate in the jungles of the wild are all too often totally inappropriate in the jungles of the boardroom or the bedroom, and although an argument with a boss or spouse may cause the sympathetic system to instinctively react, social conditioning forces us to assert cerebral dominance and act in ways that totally deny our roiling guts.

When acted out, the fight or flight response

leads to a deep parasympathetic rebound that ultimately leaves the ANS balanced. If cerebrally inhibited, sympathetic dominance remains unresolved and though we behave in a civilized manner, the base brain, and its visceral components, remain primed for action. It is this lack of resolution that leads to the initiation of the GAS and its degenerative consequences.

The problem is further compounded by the fact that, in lieu of acting upon our instincts and initiating a concomitant parasympathetic rebound, creating autonomic balance is a learned response requiring skill and patience. Autonomic balance does not occur merely with the cessation of activity; in other words, sitting down in front of the TV after a stressful day at the office will not relieve the neuroendocrinologically mediated knot in your belly. In this culture, with its constant bombardment of sensory stimuli and emphasis on doing and achieving, the passive-receptive skills necessary to engender autonomic balance are hard to gain indeed.[21]

This is one of the areas wherein BodyWork Shiatsu is so valuable. By directly addressing autonomic balance and clearing peripheral neural static, BodyWork Shiatsu affects chronic stress by providing a very direct biofeedback about conditions within our bodies. Recent research at the Menninger Foundation has shown that autonomic functions, once thought to be outside of conscious control, can be consciously regulated if the cerebral cortex can get consistent, reliable feedback on the conditions involved.[22] The pinpoint awareness brought to the tissues by each application of pressure allows the cerebral cortex to become aware of specific local conditions in the myofascial and reflex networks, an awareness not normally available to consciousness. By paying careful attention to these sensations, and by consciously relaxing and breathing through the pressure, the person being treated can encourage a much deeper level of release by creating the environment necessary for the brain to alter the tissue resting-length pattern stored in the medulla. By reeducating the neuromuscular programs stored in the brain, the effects of treatment are integrated in a much more lasting fashion.

Sympathetic dominance, the underlying neurological "cause" of stress, is experienced as a kind of static in the mind. This manifests as the incessant verbal dialogue that is always going on to our great distraction. In the body this excess manifests as the facilitated segments of the nervous system, which are the hidden force behind many of the chronic aches and pains that seem to continue without any visible cause of support.

I conjecture that because of the intensity of the stimulation of BodyWork Shiatsu on the nervous system, the sensory overload conveyed to the brain serves to clear the static from the lines, much like blowing out a clogged pipe. This is the causitive mechanism behind the ability of BodyWork Shiatsu to create a very quiet state of mind. The intensity of afferent stimulation to the spinal cord during a BodyWork Shiatsu treatment results in a general lowering of the energetic level of the internuncial neural pool. As a result, facilitated segments of the spinal cord return to normal activity, as do the overly excited tissues they innervate. This relaxation is evidenced by the palpably increased pliability of the spine after treatment.

Neuro-histologically, the intensity of stimulation promotes the synthesis of enkephalins in the body and endorphins in the brain. These naturally occurring, opiatelike neuropeptides, which act as neurotransmitters, dramatically reduce chronic pain and create a euphoric post-treatment state that can last for many hours. In combination with those techniques that directly inhibit overactivity of the sympathetic nervous system and recreate autonomic balance, the release of these neuropeptides has profound consequences in the treatment of stress.

The act of paying concentrated attention for an extended period of time effectively turns the experience of receiving BodyWork Shiatsu into a form of meditation, bringing additional benefits in terms of dealing with stress.

STRAINS AND SPRAINS

Soft-tissue injuries can be divided into two categories according to the specific tissues involved: strains are injuries to musculo-tendinous units, while sprains are soft tissue injuries involving joints. *Sprain* is defined as "The forcible wrenching or twisting of a joint with partial rupture or other injury to its attachments without luxation. There may be damage to the associated blood vessels, muscles, tendons, ligaments, or nerves."[23] Sprains usually result in ligament laxity and the formation of adhesions. While adhesions can be treated, I do not know of effective bodywork techniques to correct stretched ligaments. The pecking technique in acupuncture is said to help; proliferant injections of solutions that stimulate fibroblasts to begin laying down new collagen fibers that shorten and strengthen the ligaments is a technique that is helpful, but it must be done by a physician and requires great precision to be effective.[24]

Strain is defined as "Trauma to the muscle or musculotendinous unit from violent contraction or excessive forcible stretch. May be associated with failure of synergistic action of muscles."[25] Strains always have two components: the myofascial and the neuromuscular. Myofascial trauma results from myological or fascial microtearing, where the myofibrils of a muscle bundle or collagen fibers of fascial tissue are ruptured by traumatic insult. When myofascial tissues are ruptured they immediately exude a sticky, viscous fluid to fill the intercellular spaces of the traumatized tissues. The immediate effect of this emergency first aid is the formation of a buffering bandage that prevents the torn tissue from further trauma and causes the severed ends of the separated tissues to be held in close approximation, thus facilitating the healing process.

While necessary and effective as emergency first aid, the body is subsequently unable to dissolve the hardened exudate. This often results in pathological consequences, as fibers are not only bound end to end but also to adjacent tissues; thus, separate tissues may adhere to each other. These adhesions represent one of the causes for the increasing inflexibility and loss of mobility in aging bodies. The ability to individually contract muscles is necessary for free range of motion and efficient use of energy. Adhesive glueing forces collateral and antagonist muscles into contraction in concert with the prime movers of any specific action. This extra muscular effort, in activities that do not require the active support of these accessory muscular groups, constantly and unnecessarily squanders energy and restricts free movement. Without intervention this condition can endure for life.

Myofascial injuries respond well to hand-healing techniques. Digital compression transforms the matrix material that forms the ground substance of all connective tissues from its normally turgid gel state to the malleable sol state. Cross-fiber friction, called *kenbiki* in Japanese, is able to free adhered myofibrils and collagen fibers, restoring unimpeded movement to restricted tissues. By utilizing these techniques, even scar tissue of long-standing duration can be mobilized.

The neuromuscular component of strain injuries involves an entirely different pathomechanism. Osteopath Dr. Lawrence Jones postulates that when a muscle goes from extreme extension into sudden contraction due to startle or trauma, the involved muscle spindles become hyperfacilitated, switching in an instant from a state where they are reporting no information at all to one in which they are firing furiously. These muscle spindles continue to send signals to the brain indicating a too-rapid shortening long after the initiating movement has ended. This results in cortical interpretation of the neutral position of the involved joint as one of overextension, and results in chronic hypercontraction of the muscle as the brain tries, unsuccessfully, to shut down the inappropriate strain signal generated by the facilitated muscle spindle.

A vicious cycle ensues, with chronic hypertonicity of the myofascial tissues and resulting ischemia causing increased neural irritation and hyperfacilitation, increased muscular contraction, and so on. This not only leads to the fibrous degradation of the involved muscle, but causes deranged balance of the joints spanned by the activated muscle, which produces a concomitant effect on the antagonist and collateral muscles and also on the neural capsule of the involved joint.[26]

The nervous system lacks an inherent mechanism for resetting such hyperfacilitated proprioceptors, and so such a condition can endure for life, resulting in chronic strains being inappropriately activated over and over by stressors that would normally be insufficient to cause an injury. The chronic bad ankle, back, and so on has led both the medical and athletic communities to view myofascial strains as more pernicious than fractures, which normally heal pain-free and stronger than before the break.

This neuromuscular component of strains can be more intractable than the myofascial component, depending on the duration of the injury. But digital compression to the appropriate trigger points (i.e., the facilitated muscle spindles) results in their neutralization. Equally effective, and less painful, is the osteopathic technique of counterstrain, called positional release or orthobionomy by the bodywork community. Utilizing this approach, the affected muscles or joints are positioned exactly to the posture of maximum comfort, usually mimicking the original position from which the strain was initiated. This allows the central nervous system to gradually turn down the "gain" on the hyperfacilitated proprioceptors, allowing for the return to easy neutral of the involved tissues.[27] It is my experience that the appropriate application of digital compression facilitates the neurological rebalancing that occurs in the position of release, greatly speeding this rehabilitative process.

CHRONIC PAIN

In addition to increasing the production of enkephalins and endorphins, BodyWork Shiatsu is effective in relieving chronic pain by breaking the pain–spasm–pain cycle. Sprains, strains, crushes, and tearing injuries always lead to a contraction in the surrounding myofascial tissues. This contracture or splinting of the myofascia is one of the first aid measures the body employs to protect the site of injury from increased trauma. In conjunction with adhesive glueing, these first aid measures can lead to the establishment of a pain–spasm–pain cycle, and subsequent chronic pain, long after the acute trauma has healed.

Any constriction in the tissue will cause stagnation in the flow of the various bodily fluids coursing through that tissue, and the resultant ischemia and buildup of metabolic wastes is itself a cause of further insult to the site of trauma. In addition, I conjecture that the bio-electric fields flowing through the injury form whirlpools of static charge in these contracted muscles. This electromagnetic static exists reciprocally with the contracted muscles. Stasis strengthens contraction, and contraction feeds stasis.

The problem is compounded by the secondary side effects of the excess free radicals generated at the site of injury in this process. These are the real cause of the soreness that develops around the trauma a day or two later. In addition to the malnutritive and irritating conditions thus engendered, the contracted myofascial tissue constantly compresses the very nerves handling communication about the injury. This combination of causes leads to the establishment of the pain–spasm–pain cycle, a primary mechanism in the genesis of chronic pain.

While the healthy body enjoys a vital and effective emergency medical service, the cleanup and repair teams of the body are not so efficient. As a consequence, the body is strewn with littered memorials to the battles of life. Regardless of how the cycle is broken, once out of this destructive feedback loop the body can handle healing its component parts. It is by breaking the pain aspect of the cycle that the allopathic approach of prescribing pain killers and muscle relaxants works.

BodyWork Shiatsu creates a hyperemic rebound that flushes out toxic residues and brings a rush of fresh arterial blood to treated tissues. It proprioceptively lengthens myofascial tissues, relieving entrapped nerves, and electrochemically and mechanically frees adhesions, thus breaking the cycle of the pain–spasm–pain syndrome simultaneously in multiple systems.

THE OCEAN OF MOVEMENT

From our phylogenetic evolution as single cell organisms in the oceans of the earth, through the neonatal amniotic ocean that sustains our personal development, to the tidal respiratory, circulatory, and craniosacral rhythms of our inner environment, movement provides the central core of our experience of life. Constant enough to be placed as background to the central "I" of our personal identity, the pulsating rhythms of our inner and outer environments are an unceasing factor of physical existence. From an electromagnetic perspective, vibration—its rate, amplitude, and rate of change—are the qualities of wave motion that we can distinguish with assurance.

Based on compression as the primary technique for re-creating balance, BodyWork Shiatsu is biased toward the active Yang polarity of *doing*. The introduction of a gentle, oscillatory background to the more invasive aspects of compressive therapy, taught at the intermediate level of Body-Work Shiatsu training, offers a passive oceanic experience of the Yin pole of rhythmic movement, creating a counterbalancing effect to compressive techniques.

Rhythmic oscillation as the background for BodyWork Shiatsu creates several major effects. Constant rocking stimulates the production of an alpha state in brainwave function that augments and supports the autonomic shift from sympathetic dominance to autonomic balance. It also offers constant tactile communication throughout the intermittent applications of compression, maintaining communication and fostering deeper states of release and relaxation in the client. This continuity allows for increased surrender to the unfolding treatment, and acts as a transition stroke in BodyWork Shiatsu much as effleurage does in Swedish massage technique.

Another major benefit of oscillatory movement is its dual effect in evaluation and release. Because rhythmic movement is central to our physical experience, gentle oscillation is experienced as a comforting, noninvasive entrance into the somatic complex. Flowing from low amplitude, long-period rocking to more energetic jostling, the therapist can easily identify, evaluate, and treat myofascial, energetic, and joint restrictions with-

out challenging the protective splinting mechanisms that are easily provoked by compression.

Joints, the intrinsic muscles that cross over them, and the outermost sleeve of extrinsic muscle are all innervated by the same nerve root. Somatic dysfunction, whether at the level of the joint, the core, or the sleeve, will produce a reciprocal dysfunction in the complementary components.

From an Oriental energetic viewpoint, a restriction in Qi flow, whether deep or superficial, will over time result in the restricted flow of Qi through the entire region. In electromagnetic terms, the restriction of neuro-electromembranous circulation created by myofascial contracture at any level results in the formation of a static charge or field in the area of restriction, resulting in impeded field dynamics at every level.

While free energetic flow can certainly be reestablished by the neuroionic and electromembraneous techniques of acupuncture and Body-Work Shiatsu, it is time-consuming and often wearisome. By initiating movement at the level of restriction, the static field can be immediately interrupted. At that point, myofascial contractures can be easily corrected by BodyWork Shiatsu techniques.

When dysfunction lies in the region of joint articulation, an oscillatory movement, produced by gently and rhythmically rotating the articulating joint segments in opposing directions, serves to immediately free articular movement, breaking up intrinsic contracture and the subsequent splinting of the extrinsic sleeve. When the dysfunction is in the extrinsic myofascia, the same result is generated by jostling the contracted tissues, which the therapist accomplishes by grasping the tissues with both hands and mobilizing the myofascia in a rhythmical, opposing, back and forth movement. I have termed these combined procedures *jostlation*, recognizing that application of either oscillation or jostling will depend on the location of contracture. The important aspect of this technique has to do with the fact that, once the static field is broken, myofascial contractures melt under digital compression quickly, easily, and painlessly. While enabling the therapist to identify areas of congestion, rhythmic movements simultaneously perform an active therapeutic role, distracting the bodymind away from the splinting reflex of over-loaded sensory nerve pathways and neutralizing chronic muscular contractions. Deeper and more sustained compression becomes acceptable due to the decrease in the pain–spasm–pain cycle, thus facilitating the effectiveness of compressive therapy. From an energetic standpoint, congested Qi is encouraged to return to its normal flowing condition, and the work of freeing Qi flow, or relaxing tense muscles, is greatly facilitated.

PART 3

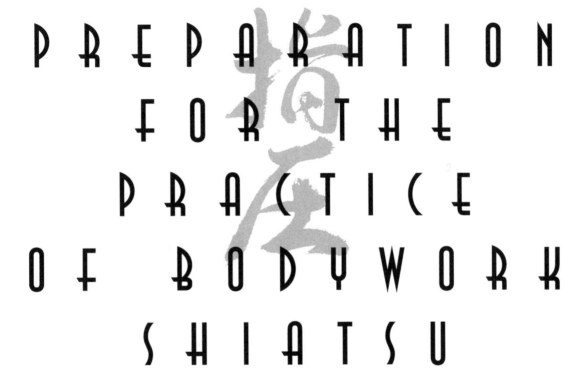

PREPARATION FOR THE PRACTICE OF BODYWORK SHIATSU

CHAPTER 7

FINGER AND HAND TECHNIQUES

I N   T H I S   C H A P T E R   W E   W I L L   address a number of theoretical and practical considerations about giving a BodyWork Shiatsu treatment. Although the technique described in this book constitutes a basic full-body treatment aimed at stimulating the flow of Qi throughout the body, this information relates equally to the more advanced, therapeutic levels of BodyWork Shiatsu practice as well.

PROPRIOCEPTION

The peripheral components of the nervous system are categorized according to the parts of the body that they innervate. The pattern of innervation is determined in utero, and corresponds to the original three layers of embryological tissue.

1. *Exteroceptors* innervate ectodermal tissue, which covers the surface of the body.
2. *Proprioceptors* innervate mesodermal tissue, which forms the muscles and joints.

3. *Interoceptors* innervate internal organs formed from the endoderm.

The competent practice of BodyWork Shiatsu primarily depends upon a well developed and extremely sensitive proprioceptive sense, since it is this aspect of the nervous system that is responsible for delicate, refined movement. By becoming consciously aware of the proprioceptive feedback taking place within our own bodies, we can learn to sense the bio-electromagnetic, central, and autonomic nervous system flows within others much more quickly and precisely than would otherwise be possible.

Taber's Medical Dictionary defines *proprioception* as "The awareness of posture, movement, and changes in equilibrium, and the knowledge of position, weight, and resistance of objects in relation to the body." Proprioceptive sense is defined as "The correlation of unconscious sensations from the skin and joints that allows conscious appreciation of the position of the body."[1]

Muscle spindles, Pacinian corpuscles, Golgi

tendon organs, and labyrinthine receptors comprise the sensory receptors of the proprioceptive nervous system. While the normal integrating and controlling functions of proprioception are performed by the medulla oblongata, that portion of the base brain concerned with the regulation of autonomic functions (hence *Taber's* characterization as "unconscious sensations"), we can, through awareness and practice, develop greatly refined, conscious control of this system.[2] Disciplines such as Hanna Somatic exercises, hatha yoga, tai chi chuan, or qi kung, created within cultures that prized such sensory information, are based on developing a subtle awareness of internal proprioceptive cues. Practice of these bodymind disciplines can be an enormous aid in acquiring and honing proprioceptive sensitivity.

The practice of BodyWork Shiatsu involves subtle communication between the hands of the therapist and the body of the client. The practitioner is, in effect, attempting to override the prevailing bio-electromagnetic, central motor, and autonomic processes that are involved in the imbalances being addressed. Although much of the information we receive, and the treatment we perform, takes place on the surface of the skin, many of the effects we are actually causing are targeted toward processes taking place deep within the body. To effectively gather the information relevant to each situation, as well as to communicate desired new patterns of activity, we must receive, integrate, and transmit extremely subtle information through our hands, a task that is impossible to achieve using our normal tactile sensory channels.

For example, when dealing with adhesive contractures at the level of the intrinsic musculature, it is necessary to perceive conditions and transmit directions for change through many layers of intervening tissue. While this level of proprioceptive feedback is not normally available to ordinary awareness, it can be learned by long, patiently applied, conscious effort. Over the course of time and through much experience, every BodyWork Shiatsu therapist learns to "see" and "speak" through the hands in order to effect such delicate communication.

The bio-electromagnetic field the body generates can be measured at some distance from the skin surface; how far depends on the vital strength of the field and the sensitivity of the measuring instruments. Once a therapist's hands are placed on a client's body, their biofields are merged. It then becomes possible, so long as the therapist's intentions are in the best interest of the client—irrespective of the mechanical, neuromuscular techniques employed—for the therapist to directly influence the bio-field–mediated functions of the person being treated.

Clarity of awareness, energetic strength, concentration, and purity of intention—these are the necessary qualities of a practitioner performing a successful BodyWork Shiatsu treatment. Through utilizing well-developed proprioceptive skills, the relief we provide our clients by influencing their energetic biofield can exceed the effects of any specific massage techniques we may employ. The degree of skill acquired depends entirely upon the effort extended to master our own proprioceptive powers.

COMPLIANCE

The hand is perhaps the most evolved part of our anatomical structure. It is also the most obvious point of interaction between therapist and client. *Compliance,* as discussed in this book, refers to the ability of the hand to maintain constant, nondifferentiated contact with the part(s) of the body being treated. Our hands have the unparalleled ability to take the shape of whatever they contact; they permit us to merge boundaries with, and become part of, whatever we are holding.

The exactitude with which we can proprioceive through and micromanipulate the palmar surface of our hands is mirrored in the sensorimotor portion of our cerebral cortex. With the exception of the lips, the hands (especially the thumbs) take up the largest proportional amount of neuronal space in this region of the brain, as illustrated by the sensorimotor homunculi (figs. 7.1 and 7.2).

Not only during stationary contact, but also while our hands are moving over the constantly changing contours of our client's body, we can maintain continuous therapeutic contact with whatever tissue-phase boundary we are treating. Although inherent in the phenomenally complex anatomical structure of the human hand, this ability is only developed by the constant application of compassionate, nonjudgmental, merged touch

practiced over a long period of time. Compliance is an active demonstration of our understanding of the basic principle of unity.

The person we are treating is a unified organism made up of many overlapping and interrelated energy fields and physical structures. If we approach the moment of contact with our minds and hands already targeted for a specific objective, we miss the opportunity to respond to the immediate needs of that being. While we must use our powers of discrimination to assess energetic balance and to plan our treatment strategy, the actual moment of contact requires being in "beginner's mind" if we are to truly perceive, and appropriately respond to, the conditions we are addressing.

The refined proprioceptive skill of compliance requires detachment and distance from our own superficial sensory apparatus. The entire body must be brought into play. Information must be gathered and integrated from the initial stage of visual assessment, through the subtle experience of

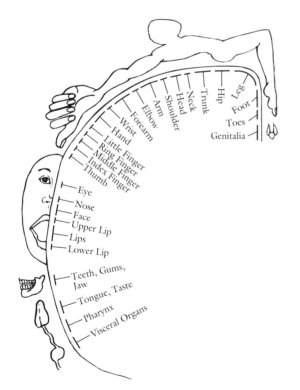

Fig. 7.1. The Sensory Cortex Homunculus

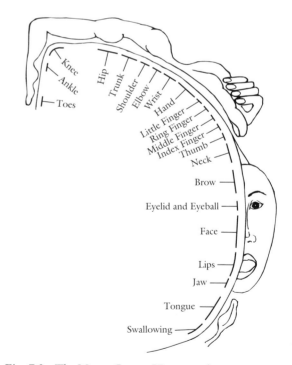

Fig. 7.2. The Motor Cortex Homunculus

biofield interaction, to the moment of physical contact and beyond.

Soft hands filled with energy and life, responsive to the needs of each moment, strong yet gentle—these are the qualities of compliance. Compliant hands may be directed to whatever level of the client's body is calling out for treatment. When this skill is mastered, specific techniques become secondary to therapeutic intent. Therapist and client are one. Trust and comfort surround this interaction. At this place the Great Healer is made welcome.

COMPRESSION

In this book *compression* refers to the technique of applying pressure to the human body. Pressure may be applied with the fingers, fingertips, thumbs, palms, edge of the hands, knuckles, forearms, elbows, knees, or feet. It may be gentle or deep, reaching to many different levels; it may be steady or intermittent; it may be applied gradually or suddenly; or it may be a combination of any of these elements.

The specific compression technique employed is always determined by the condition of the body and the effects you desire to create. Each situation is unique; the same technique can produce many different effects, depending on the circumstances. Gentle, brief, steady pressure is generally tonifying (stimulating), while hard, deep, long pressure applied irregularly is sedating. For general tonification, which is the level of practice being taught in this book, pressure should be applied gently to the desired depth and in one even movement. The compression is held for the required length of time

and smoothly released. Jerky, uneven movement should be avoided.

CYLINDERS

Because the human body presents so many uneven contours, we will consider each section of the body that is to be treated as a cylinder. In a BodyWork Shiatsu treatment, pressure is always directed perpendicular to the point of compression. For example, if the erector spinae muscle group is viewed as a cylinder, then pressure is always directed toward the center of the cylinder (see fig. 7.3). In this instance the medial border of the erector spinae cylinder is pressed at a 45-degree angle lateral, toward the center of the imaginary cylinder formed by the muscle group. The Bladder 1 (Bl1) meridian, running through the center of the erector spinae muscle group (1½ acu-inches from the spinous process)* receives pressure directly downward. The Bl2 meridian, running through the lateral margin of the erector spinae cylinder, is pressed at a 45-degree angle medial, toward the center of the cylinder. Thus, despite the apparent superficial direction, pressure is always oriented toward the center of the underlying cylinder.

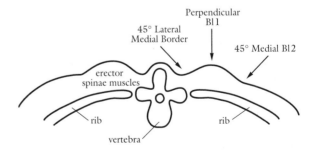

Fig. 7.3. Angle of Pressure

---

* An acu-inch is a variable unit of measurement derived proportionally from the specific area being treated. In general, an acu-inch is equal to the space between the second and third interphalangeal lines of the middle finger.

The finger pressure employed in the basic BodyWork Shiatsu treatment is generally tonifying, and always within the comfort range of the recipient. For greatest effectiveness and ease of performance, finger pressure should:

- Be firm and steady, without vibration or circular friction;
- Be directed toward the center of the pathway cylinder;
- Be derived from the coordination of weight and gravity, rather than by muscular power.

USE OF THE FINGERS AND THUMBS

In this general BodyWork Shiatsu treatment, either the pad of the thumb overlying the central swirl of the fingerprint or the full length of the thumb is used, depending on the area of the body being worked. Since this level of treatment is essentially meant to stimulate the body's vital functions, deep penetrating pressure is not necessary. On the broader portions of the back, the pad of the thumb is most frequently used; on the neck and limbs, the entire thumb; on the abdomen, the fingers and fingertips and the palm and heel of the hand. The broad, gentle pressure thus generated ensures the client's comfort and also provides proper stimulation of the pathway Qi. Figure 7.4 shows the parts of the fingers and hand referred to in the treatment instructions. Figure 7.5 illustrates some of the hand positions we will be using in our practice of BodyWork Shiatsu.

To perform digital compressions without causing undue irritation by "nailupuncture," the nails must be kept very short. Just beyond the bed of the nail is the length that will best protect both therapist and client. Shorter nails will be painful and

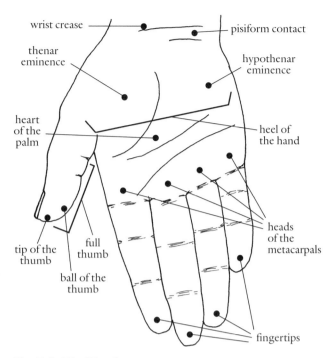

Fig. 7.4. The Hand

longer nails will restrict finger use. The line of cut should be fairly straight, leaving a support at the medial and lateral edges rather than a curve following the nail bed. Needless to say, the nails must be filed smooth of rough edges.

If you are used to having longer nails, this type of nail care may initially provoke some discomfort in the form of fingertip sensitivity and loss of dexterity. But it will, in a very short time, result in more effective use of the tools of your craft. The initial sensitivity of the flesh around the nail bed lessens with time, and the tissue itself changes. Protective pads, or caps, will form all around the fingertips. This toughened flesh will help you as a bodywork therapist. As well, the initial loss of dexterity due to the absence of nails (think of how often nails are used to pry or scrape) is rapidly restored by the heightened proprioceptive skills developed by the practice of BodyWork Shiatsu. In time, unclipped nails will become a distraction, interfering with the action of truly sensitized fingertips.

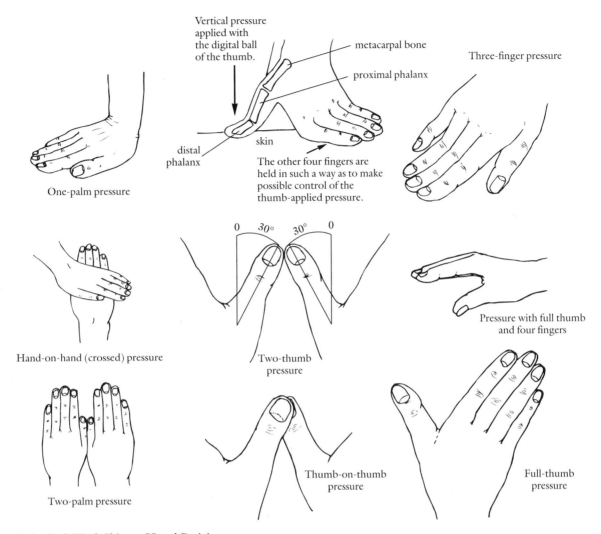

Fig. 7.5. *BodyWork Shiatsu Hand Positions*

One-palm pressure

Vertical pressure applied with the digital ball of the thumb.

metacarpal bone

proximal phalanx

distal phalanx

skin

The other four fingers are held in such a way as to make possible control of the thumb-applied pressure.

Three-finger pressure

Hand-on-hand (crossed) pressure

0   30°   30°   0

Two-thumb pressure

Pressure with full thumb and four fingers

Two-palm pressure

Thumb-on-thumb pressure

Full-thumb pressure

Hygiene

A word about hygiene: hand, finger, and nail cleanliness is essential for the professional practice of BodyWork Shiatsu, not only because clients are repelled by dirty hands, but also because dirt and oil form a kind of insulation, blocking the reception and transmission of subtle body energies. Hands should be washed with soap and warm water before and after every treatment, then rinsed with cold water up to the elbow after every session. You should also shake out your hands after working on someone. This will protect you from the many different kinds of impurities and imbalances that you might pick up from your clients during a treatment.

These hygienic practices are essential in order to protect yourself. Unless you are in a state of radiant vital health, you can easily absorb distorted energies from your client. Your best defense is the regular preventive practice of Qi-enhancing and Qi-circulating practices. Keeping your own Qi abundant and free flowing is the best way to maintain your vital health. Nevertheless, it is prudent to shake off any polluted electromagnetic charge left in your arms after treatment, preferably out of sight of your client, and to rinse your hands and lower arms thoroughly with cold water. This procedure produces a clearly felt sense of cleanliness on many levels.[3]

CHAPTER 8

ROAD SIGNS

THE STANDARD MEDICAL terminology used to describe directions in the body is shown in Figure 8.1. These terms will be used throughout the following chapters.

Anterior	Toward the front of the body
Posterior	Toward the back of the body
Cephalad	Toward the head
Caudal	Toward the feet
Lateral	From the midline out
Medial	Toward the centerline
Superior	Above
Inferior	Below

STANDARD LINES

Standard lines are used as guides for locating specific acupoints, meridians, or other anatomical landmarks in order to apply BodyWork Shiatsu techniques. The standard lines as described below are illustrated in figures 8.2 through 8.4. These lines are of special value when the normal bony contours of the body are obscured by excess flesh, or your therapeutic target area is inside the body as opposed to being on the surface.

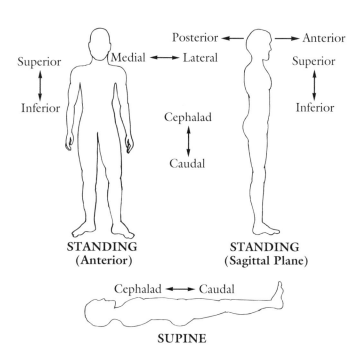

Fig. 8.1. Directions in the Body

Posterior Torso

POSTERIOR HORIZONTAL LINES

There are four horizontal lines on the posterior torso (fig. 8.2).

1. Line one runs between C7 and T1, the two largest spinous processes at the cervicothoracic juncture. (To distinguish between the two, flex the neck and rotate the head from side to side; C7 is the spinous process that moves.)

2. Line two runs along the inferior border of the scapulae in anatomical position, at the level of T7. (In the "ideal" body, the scapulae lie between the second and seventh thoracic vertebrae. When the client is lying prone, the scapulae ride up higher on the thorax; to locate the second standard line they must be depressed in a caudal direction.)

3. Line three passes across the lowermost border of the rib cage, at the tips of the eleventh ribs, level with the twelfth thoracic vertebra. This line marks the inferolateral border of the respiratory diaphragm, the middle of the three transverse fascial restrictions of the torso.[1]

4. Line four lies across the crest of the ilia. Because of anatomical differences, this line falls between the third and fourth lumbar vertebrae on a man and at the fifth lumbar vertebra on a woman.

POSTERIOR VERTICAL LINES

There are four vertical lines also to be found on the posterior torso (fig. 8.2).

1. Line one runs down the center of the spinous processes.
2. Line two lies $\frac{1}{2}$ acu-inch bilateral to the

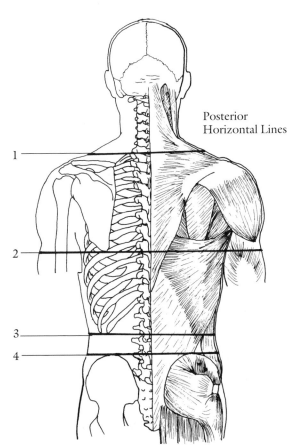

Posterior Horizontal Lines

Fig. 8.2. Posterior Lines

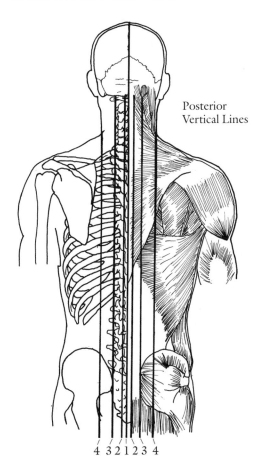

Posterior Vertical Lines

4 3 2 1 2 3 4

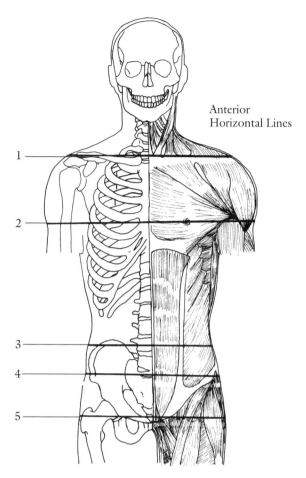

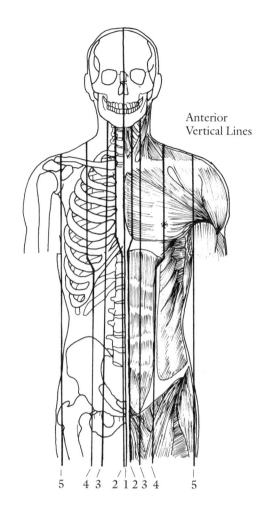

Fig. 8.3. Anterior Lines

spine, along the medial margins of the erector spinae muscles.

3. Line three lies 1½ acu-inches lateral to the spinous processes, in the middle of the erector spinae cylinder.

4. Line four lies 1½ acu-inches lateral to the third lines, on the lateral margin of the erector spinae cylinder.

Anterior Torso

ANTERIOR HORIZONTAL LINES

There are five horizontal lines on the anterior torso (fig. 8.3).

1. Line one lies across the thoracic inlet; it crosses the point where the heads of the clavicles articulate with the sternum. The

locomotive, circulatory, neurological, craniosacral, respiratory, and nutrient transport systems all communicate between the brain and the body through this passageway. This region constitutes the most superior of the three transverse fascial restrictions of the torso.

2. Line two passes through the nipple line, between the fourth and fifth ribs. The location of this line must be approximated on women.

3. Line three passes through the umbilicus, overlying the fourth lumbar vertebra.

4. Line four runs through the anterior superior iliac crests (ASIS), level with the base of the sacrum.

5. Line five runs across the top of the pubic bone, overlying the pelvic diaphragm.

This is the most caudal of the three transverse fascial restrictions of the torso.

ANTERIOR VERTICAL LINES

There are also five vertical lines on the anterior torso (fig. 8.3).

1. Line one runs along the ventral midline, passing through the linea alba and the centerline of the sternum.
2. Line two runs bilaterally along the medial border of the rectus abdominis, ½ acu-inch lateral to the midline. At the xiphoid process it veers laterally to follow the lateral borders of the sternum to the heads of the clavicles.
3. Line three runs through the middle of the rectus abdominis muscle 2 acu-inches lateral to the midline, crossing the inferior border of the rib cage at the sixth rib. It then passes up the thorax halfway between the midline and the nipple line.
4. Line four runs up the lateral margin of the rectus abdominis muscle, veering lateral at the base of the rib cage to ascend vertically through the nipple line.
5. Line five runs through the anterior axillary crease.

LATERAL VERTICAL LINE

The lateral vertical line runs from the cranial vertex through the centerline of the ear, the lateral aspect of the head of the humerus, the center of the axillary space, the greater trochanter of the femur, the head of the fibula, and the lateral malleolus of the ankle (fig. 8.4).

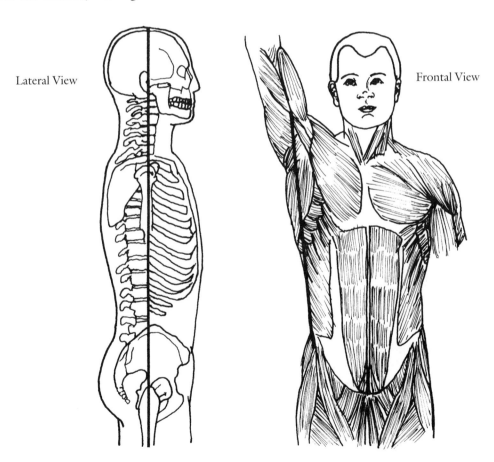

Lateral View

Frontal View

Fig. 8.4. Lateral Vertical Line

Additional Anatomical Landmarks

- The tip of the twelfth rib lies at the level of the second lumbar vertebra (L2).
- To find the twelfth thoracic vertebra, place two or three fingers on the iliac crest. Palpate in an upward direction with your thumb until you feel the inferior margin of the twelfth rib. Then run your fingers toward each other, lightly and quickly, in the diagonal line indicated by the ribs. An alternate method is to palpate the lateral edge of the eleventh rib; the body of the twelfth thoracic vertebra is in that horizontal plane.
- The suprasternal notch, the area above the manubrium and between the heads of the clavicles, lies at the level of the second thoracic vertebra (T2).
- The sternal angle, the area between the second and third ribs, lies at the level of the fourth thoracic vertebra (T4).
- The xiphoid process, located at the inferior tip of the sternum, lies at the level of the ninth thoracic vertebra (T9).

CHAPTER 9

AT YOUR TABLE

FOR THOUSANDS OF YEARS Oriental bodywork has been practiced on a futon on the floor, and throughout the first eight years of my practice that was how I worked. Then, following arthroscopic knee surgery to correct old injuries, I transferred my treatment to a massage table.

What a revolution! My creaky knees ceased to limit the number of treatments I could give each day. I found that by utilizing stances I had learned in practicing martial arts, I could use my legs instead of my lower back to support my body weight. By employing these stances when treating the client on a table, my finger pressure flowed naturally from gravity rather than muscle power. Working in this way conserved my energy and allowed the client's body to intuitively understand and cooperate with my finger pressure, letting the treatment penetrate deeply. I was easily able to add one more session to each workday.

Older clients as well as severely injured ones began to call me for appointments. These were people who had heard about my work but were put off by the thought of having to get on the floor for treatments. All in all, my practice increased by about 30 percent after I switched to a table.

Subsequently I've discovered that all clinical practice in China takes place on sturdy, low tables, or on chairs. In Japan some traditional practitioners still work on a futon, but most clinical practice is now performed on a table as well.

THE TABLE

The table you choose is a decision of major importance. If you are not working exclusively in a clinic, or at home, your table must be light and portable to facilitate an out-call practice. The table must also be sturdy enough to hold two people—you must be able to get on and off of the table easily as you work on different parts of your client's body. Appearance and comfort are additional considerations. It's a joy to have a professionally crafted table, and needless to say, comfort is critical, especially if your practice includes older or seriously injured clients. Select a table that is comfortable to lie on for an hour with little or no movement.

Although making a portable table is much less expensive than buying one, the difference in craftsmanship, handleability, comfort, and professional appearance make this a poor choice. Several companies make excellent portable tables.

Because you must work at different heights to treat different parts of the body, your table must allow you to do so without distorting your posture. I find that the best general height is to have the top of the table reach my palms when the wrists are flexed and the arms are extended toward my feet. This height allows me to treat limbs by deepening my stance, yet it still permits easy access to the back or abdomen. Whatever the table height, it must allow you to focus your pressure from the center of your hara, the point called dan tien, located 1½ inches below the navel.

In order to emulate the body mechanics of working on the floor, the table must be wide enough to easily accommodate you and your client as you kneel on the table while treating the back. A width of thirty-three inches is optimal. A more narrow table causes the practitioner to teeter on the edge; a wider table requires bending to reach the client while working from a standing position.

The padding on your table must be thick enough to insure comfort yet firm enough to allow you to work deeply. The padding must also protect your knees from discomfort when you kneel on the table. The seams on the edges and corners of your table should be smooth, with no loose flaps or protruding parts. To protect your knees I recommend at least one inch of high-density foam covered with at least two inches of medium density foam. This padding gives the table a luxurious feel.

Accessories

Chairs

The use of chairs for the treatment of arm, shoulder, neck, face, and cranial problems is common in clinical settings throughout the Orient. Seated treatment is a traditional aspect of Oriental bodywork. Any straight-backed chair is suitable, as long as the height allows you to work from your center of gravity, and the back of the chair does not interfere with the area you are treating.

The growing practice of on-site massage has resulted in the invention of elaborate portable massage chairs. These chairs vary greatly in cost, quality, and utility, but I have found several very good versions now available on the market. The good ones allow the client to sit comfortably supported in a semiprone, stable position that allows the practitioner great access to the entire back, neck, head, and arms. These chairs are easy to set up, attractive, and a great sales aid since they attract the attention of passersby. While they offer excellent support to the client, they can be awkward to use if they are not the right height for you.

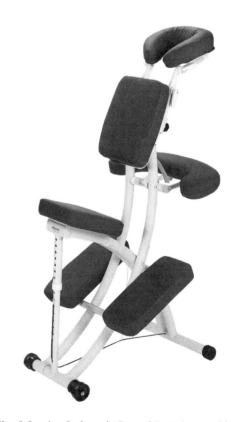

*Fig. 9.1. An Oakworks Portal Pro*2 portable massage chair.*

FACE CRADLES

Face-cradle technology has evolved greatly in the past few years. You can now buy face cradles that store under your table and adjust in all directions. Molded to allow your client to breathe, the new ones don't even leave a cradle crease on your client's face. A good cradle is a must for the added range it brings to cervical work. Be sure to get one that adjusts up and down, as well as tilting, to accommodate large-chested clients.

BOLSTERS

The use of appropriate bolsters greatly enhances client comfort during extended periods of lying still. While treating clients in a supine position, I usually place a three-inch neck roll under the cervical spine. This serves to prevent posterior cervical and cervico-cranial tension. I also use a bolster six to nine inches thick and twenty-seven inches long under the knees to insure sufficient flexion of the leg. This flexion serves to relax and flatten the lumbar curve and prevents hyperextension of the popliteal fossa.

While treating clients in a prone position, I use the same six- to nine-inch bolster under the ankles. This increased height insures comfort for the ankles, feet, and toes. It also allows for complete extension at the inguinal fold, which helps in freeing the iliolumbar and deep gluteal myofascia.

A special bolster called a bodyCushion is now available from Body Support Systems. Because the bodyCushion is contoured to the body and extraordinarily adjustable, I use it with every client when treating in the prone position. It can be used on the floor or table, and provides the most comfort and support of any system I have so far experienced.

MISCELLANEOUS

If your practice includes on-site calls, a table cover will keep your table clean and free from nicks and tears. You can get covers made to your size specifications, with built-in pockets for whatever accessories you need to carry. Wheels, either built into your cover or on a skate that straps to your table, are also essential if you want to enjoy your last session of the day as much as your first. A new product called a table carrier, built like a heavy-duty luggage carrier, is also available and is even more useful.

DRAPING

A BodyWork Shiatsu treatment may be given through cotton clothing, though I find that direct contact on the skin provides my hands the greatest degree of sensitivity. I have my clients leave their underpants on. Men are otherwise naked; my female clients wear hospital gowns open at the back. This combination provides direct access to the skin while allowing me to effectively address the issue of modesty. Although the gown interferes somewhat with abdominal treatment on women, it has proved an acceptable clinical compromise over the years. Such a compromise may not be necessary for women treating women—or even for men treating women for whom nudity is not a problem. I prefer to have all women clients wear a gown. Draping techniques that are used in oil-based massage are also fine.

STANCES

The three stances I've adopted from tai chi chuan—the Balanced Stance, the Front Stance, and the Back Stance—keep the torso balanced over the legs as you work. Specifically, these stances keep the weight of your body focused in your legs rather than in your back. In order to efficiently convert gravity into pressure, your feet must make firm and complete contact with the ground. The weight of the body must be entirely held up by the legs, the part of the body designed to support our weight. Due to unresolved physical and emotional trauma, and lacking training in proper body mechanics, most of us hold our bodies upright by contracting the muscles of the torso and shoulder girdle. This habit of carrying ourselves by the muscles of the upper body, rather than by the appropriate structural support provided by the legs, is energy-wasting and inefficient. With the torso distorted by muscular tension, gravity is unable to flow through our energetic center, and finger pressure therefore requires effort. This way of using the body is physically tiring; prolonged stress of this kind can easily lead to repetitive motion disorders in all of the major joints of the body.

Tai chi practice teaches you to keep the torso absolutely straight and balanced on the pelvis. The body is entirely supported, and moved, by the legs. This allows you to transmit force from dan tien. Pressure is applied by dropping your weight more deeply into the feet, sinking into the earth rather than leaning into your client. By always keeping the energy of dan tien focused through your hands as you apply pressure, you become an intermediary of the universe. By converting the gravitational lever of the Heavens into finger pressure upon the fulcrum of the Earth, you will never hurt yourself. Making use of these stances will allow you to enjoy your practice of BodyWork Shiatsu for a lifetime.

The designation of "opened" or "closed" in relation to stances refers to whether your body forms an acute or obtuse angle in relation to the body part being treated.

Balanced Stance
The Balanced Stance is the beginning posture of tai chi chuan (fig. 9.2). Stand with the feet one to

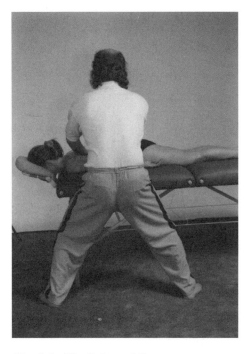
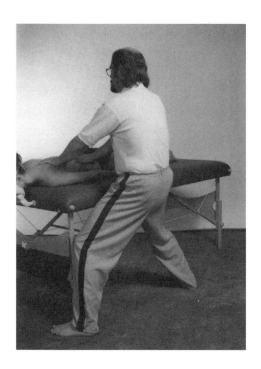

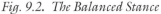
Fig. 9.2. The Balanced Stance

one and a half shoulder-widths apart and parallel, distributing the weight evenly over the bottoms of the feet so that you do not feel the weight settling in one particular area. Bend comfortably at the ankles, knees, and groin. Relax the belly, filling dan tien; relax the anus, genitals, buttocks, and the perineal area. Straighten the lower back by relaxing and rounding the lower abdomen. Drop the rib cage and float the shoulders back and down. Lower the chin slightly toward the clavicles while gently lifting and straightening the cervical vertebrae.

This tai chi posture allows the axial skeleton to balance over the bowl of the pelvis, the weight of the body being carried entirely by the legs. Movement comes from the energetic center, dan tien. With the shoulder girdle settled naturally and effortlessly on the thorax, your hands can contact the client's body in whatever manner is appropriate. Every standing BodyWork Shiatsu technique begins from this posture.

Front Stance

In the Front Stance (fig. 9.3) the legs are open in the sagittal plane (front to back), and the pelvis rotates to face directly over the front foot. The torso is resting on the pelvis, as in the Balanced Stance posture; the knees are bent enough for the ilium to stay level. The toes are about shoulder-width apart; the rear foot rotates outward to a 45-degree angle. The distance between the front and back leg depends on the technique being applied. Approximately 70 percent of your weight is on the front foot. Both feet remain flat on the ground whenever possible.

Back Stance

Maintaining the body positioning of the Front Stance, the body weight shifts onto the rear leg to rest in the Back Stance (fig. 9.4). The pelvis remains facing the front foot; the front foot is still pointing forward. As in the Balanced Stance, the torso is

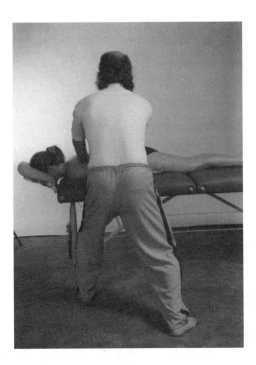

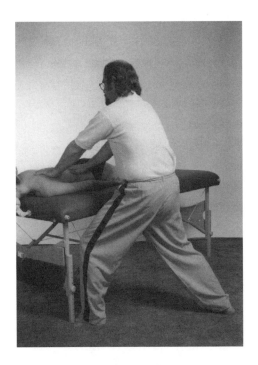

Fig. 9.3. The Front Stance

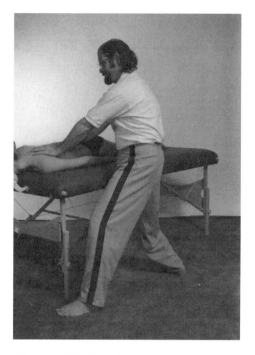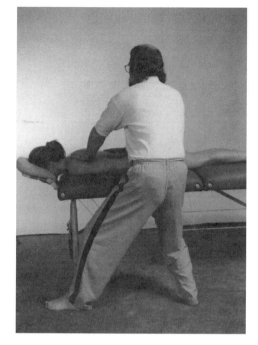

Fig. 9.4. The Back Stance

aligned over the pelvis. At least 70 percent of the body's weight is on the rear foot. The distance between the legs is determined by the technique being applied.

This completes the philosophical and theoretical basis for the practice of Oriental bodywork. The information we have covered provides you with an adequate background for the actual practice of the beginning level of BodyWork Shiatsu. Some of this information is quite different from the considerations of Western science, but it is logically coherent and has stood the test of time. Be sure to reread any material that has escaped your understanding during the first reading—you will find that it suddenly makes sense the second time through.

In the following chapters on the actual techniques of BodyWork Shiatsu, you will find it much easier to master the routines if you make an audio tape that you can play back as you practice. Read the directions slowly enough so that you can follow them easily. As you work to increase your level of skill, keep in mind the response of the master whose student asked him how to get to Carnegie Hall: "Practice, practice, practice." Good luck: sincere effort will be rewarded many hundredfold.

PART 4

FULL-
BODY
TREATMENT

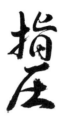

THE TREATMENT being presented in this book is a basic meridian-oriented, full-body shiatsu/anma treatment, designed for general relaxation and tonification of the entire system. Because the intent is to stimulate the flow of Qi on the surface of the body, the hand techniques we will be using are gentle and only mildly penetrating.

We usually picture shiatsu techniques as being deep and forceful, and sedative hand techniques are just that. This treatment, however, is not targeted toward any specific therapeutic goal other than enhancing the flow of Qi throughout the entire body. In order to do this you must be gentle, restraining the tendency to bear down and work deeply. That will come in the next level of practice—therapeutic shiatsu/anma. If you take the time to master meridian-level practice first, you will spare your thumbs much discomfort. You will also develop a sensitivity and refinement that will serve you well throughout your entire practice.

Although there are very few absolute contraindications to the practice of Oriental bodywork, there are certain conditions that require spe-

cial training and care in order to be safely treated or treated at all. Until you have received such training from a qualified expert, please exercise extreme caution when a client presents with the conditions listed in appendix 1. Exercise caution in treating a client immediately after they have eaten. Also avoid giving a BodyWork Shiatsu treatment when you are feeling off-centered.

One final consideration. Although detoxification reactions (mei gen reactions) are rare when treating at this level, they can sometimes happen if your client's system is very toxic, or if you work too deeply or too long. Preventive hydrotherapy should always be recommended, and a detailed discussion of a high concentration Epsom salt contrast bath is offered in appendix 2.

You will need the following definitions as you work through the treatment sections:

Splinting reflex: When myofascial tissue is injured, the tissues surrounding the injury immediately contract to protect the injured area. Splinting is an autonomic reflex, controlled from the medulla oblongata. If the splinting becomes habitual, the injured tissues literally become invisible to the sensorimotor cortex, and the contracture can endure for life. The splinting reflex is sometimes called *protective splinting*.

Extrinsic splinting: Splinting of the extrinsic myofascial envelope, which consists of the large muscles that cover the surface of the body (as opposed to the smaller intrinsic muscles that cross the joints and initiate movement).

Residual contractive splinting: Refers to the continued contracture of the tissues surrounding the injury after the injured tissues heal. Without intervention such contractures may endure for life.

Motor release points: Acupoints lying over the motor end plates of the neuromuscular junctions that innervate muscles. They affect muscle tonus.

Origin release point: Acupoints overlying the origin, or insertion, of a muscle. They affect tendon tonus.

Distractive oscillation: Rhythmically rotating the bones that form a joint in opposite directions in order to cause the intrinsic muscles of the joint to release, increasing range of motion and initiating a release in the superficial, extrinsic musculature.

First metacarpal: The thumb.

First metatarsal: The big toe.

Jostling: Alternately pushing and pulling the muscles between joints back and forth simultaneously in order to cause them to relax and lengthen.

Jostlation: A neologism referring to the movement of joints and their controlling muscles in order to produce a reduction in myofascial tonus and an increase in range of motion. This refers to the combined techniques of oscillating and jostling.

Entry-level pressure: Compression meant to gain contact with a meridian or point that is covered by superficial tissue.

Spinal/sacral pumping: Rhythmically applying your body weight and releasing it in order to create movement in the skeleton.

Compressive friction: Friction applied after first compressing the tissues.

Sawing: A form of compressive friction.

Proprioceptive cueing: Using all of the fingers or the entire hand to apply supportive pressure in order to give the brain enough feedback about your position in space to allow for exact control of your thumb during compression.

Seki Sai Sen: Japanese for "next to the bone." Refers to the lamina groove on either side of the spinous processes.

Vertebral References (C, T, L, S): In the following section references to specific vertebra are prefaced by the initial letter of the section of the spine in which they are found. Thus the cervical vertebrae are referred to as C1–C7, the thoracic vertebrae as T1–T12, the lumbar vertebrae as L1–L5, and the sacral vertebral segments as S1–S4.

CHAPTER 10

BACK WARM-UP

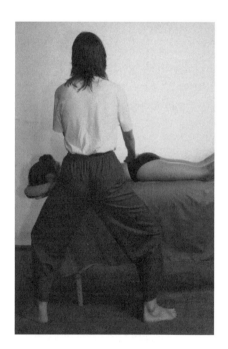

Fig. 10.1

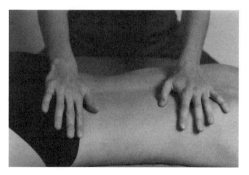

Fig. 10.2

1. Sacral Rocking

Stand at the client's left side, level with the sacrum, in a Balanced Stance (fig. 10.1). The client is lying prone on the table. Place your right palm on the sacrum and begin moving the entire pelvis with a gentle horizontal rocking motion. The pressure of your palm should be firm but not excessive and should comply to the sacrum. Find the rate and amplitude of movement that is natural for your client's body. Continue until an easeful, unrestricted rocking motion is established.

While continuing the sacral rocking with your right hand, place the heel of your left hand over the spinous processes of the lower lumbar vertebrae. Gently compress them so as to focus the rocking action at each section of the spine. Move the heel of your left hand up the spine, one palm-width at a time, to the apex of the thoracic curve (fig. 10.2) and then back down to the sacrum. Evaluate for restrictions to easeful motion. Some people will not be able to relax into this movement. If the rocking does not become easy and unrestricted after 6 to 8 repetitions, stop and move on to spinal rocking (step 2).

2. Spinal Rocking

Shifting to a caudal Front Stance, place your left hand next to your right on the spinous processes of the lower lumbar vertebrae. Initiating your movement by flexing at your ankles, begin rocking with both palms, gradually sliding your hands up the spine to the middle of the scapulae, at the apex of the thoracic curve, then back down to the sacrum (fig. 10.3). Using your body weight (not your arm strength), apply pressure through the heels of your hands to the side of the spinous processes to free any restrictions to motion. Perform spinal rocking 3 or 4 times at each position, once up and once down the spine.

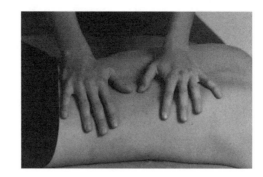

Fig. 10.3

3. Paraspinal Separation

Kneel on the table, placing your left knee below your client's left axillary space and your right knee even with the trochanter, and place your hands side by side at the base of the spine (fig. 10.4). Wedge the heels of your hands into the medial edge of the erector spinae muscle mass. Using your body weight, apply a gradually increasing lateral pressure to separate the erector spinae away from the spinous processes (fig. 10.5). Move up to the middle of the scapulae, a double hand-width at a time, and back down to the sacrum. Be careful not to apply pressure straight down, especially on clients with a history of rib injuries. (If a splinting reflex occurs, step down from the table and direct your pressure more laterally to take the pressure off the rib cage.) Maintain each compression until you feel the erector spinae muscles melting and broadening. (1 time.)

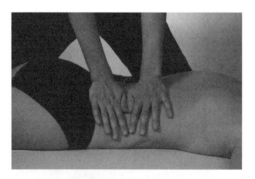

Fig. 10.4

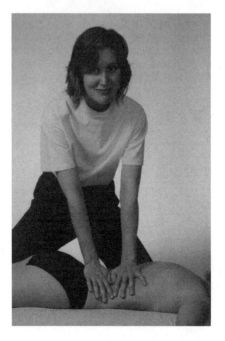

Fig. 10.5

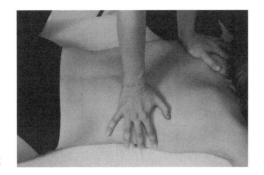

Fig. 10.6

4. Rib Mobilization and Thoracic Cross-stretch

Maintaining the same kneeling posture, place your left hand on your client's left scapula, with the hollow of your palm cupping the medial border of the scapular spine. Place your right palm on the base of the right side of the rib cage (fig. 10.6). Using your body weight, apply two-handed compression to the rib cage while stretching on a diagonal. The rib cage will compress, and the intrinsic muscles of the thoracic spine will be stretched laterally. Move your right hand up the thorax, one hand-width at a time, to the opposite scapular spine, and back to the base of the ribs. Repeat the compression and stretch at each position. Work with your client's exhalations in a rhythmic manner. Be attentive for a splinting reflex, which would indicate a prior rib injury. If a splinting reflex occurs, stop this technique and move on to the spinal cross-stretch. (1 time.)

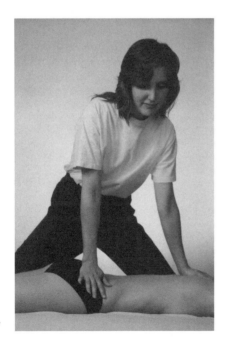

Fig. 10.7

5. Full Cross-stretch

Maintaining the same kneeling posture, place your right hand on the right sacroiliac joint, cupping the posterior superior iliac spine (PSIS) with the hollow of your palm. Leave your left hand on the left scapula, cupping the medial border of the scapular spine (fig. 10.7). Rotate your body cephalically and lean forward; shift your weight slowly onto your arms and give a diagonal stretch to the entire spine. Hold the stretch until you feel the spine release and lengthen. Be careful not to overstretch the spine. (1 time.)

**Reverse instructions and repeat
steps 2, 3, 4, and 5
on the opposite side.**

---

6. Sacral Pumping

Kneel on the table with your knees on either side of your client's left hip socket. Place the palm of your right hand in full contact with the sacrum, oriented on a longitudinal axis. The heads of your meta-carpal bones align with the sacral base, between the posterior superior iliac spines; the thenar and hypothenar eminences rest on either side of the sacral apex. Do not press on the coccyx. Your left hand lies horizontally across your right hand (fig. 10.8). Begin by tractioning the sacrum caudally to take up any slack, then pump with a torque-like twist, first to one side, then the other (fig. 10.9). Then traction the sacrum cephalically, using the same twisting pump to both sides (fig. 10.10). Use your body weight. The top hand applies the pressure while the bottom hand senses the range of motion of the sacrum. (3 times in each direction.)

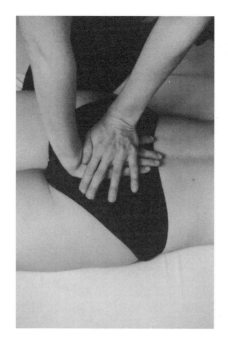

Fig. 10.8

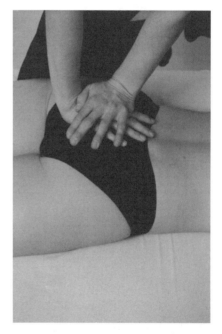

Fig. 10.9

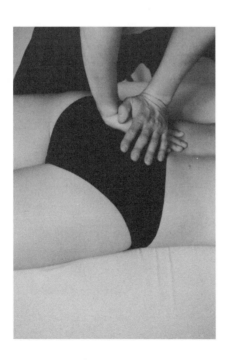

Fig. 10.10

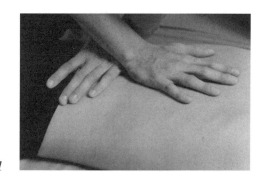

Fig. 10.11

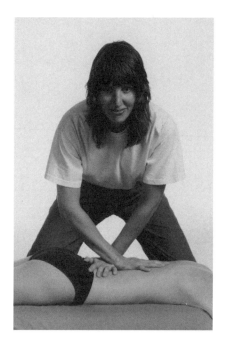

Fig. 10.12

7. Spinal Pump and Stretch

Move cephalad to kneel at the middle of the torso with your left hand resting horizontally at the top of the sacrum. Place your right hand over and next to your left hand, in longitudinal contact with the spine. The base of your right palm lies on the lower lumbar vertebrae (fig. 10.11). Rock forward over your client, using your body weight to gently depress and separate the vertebrae (fig. 10.12). As you begin to depress the spine, roll your hands apart on the pivot point of the wrists, like a can opener, in order to further separate the vertebrae. Move up the spine in two-vertebrae units to the middle of the scapular region, then back to the sacrum. Work very gently the first time, sensing for stiffness, immobility, or abnormal spinal contours. Press more firmly the second time to mobilize the interspinal myofascial tissues. (2 times.)

8. Full Cross-stretch

Maintaining the same kneeling posture, place your right hand on the right sacroiliac joint, cupping the PSIS with the hollow of your palm. Place your left hand on the left scapula, cupping the medial border of the scapular spine (fig. 10.13). Rotate your body cephalically and lean forward; shift your weight slowly onto your arms and give a diagonal stretch to the entire spine. Hold the stretch until your client releases and you feel the spine lengthen. Then open your position caudally and place your left hand on the medial border of the right scapular spine; shift your right hand to the left PSIS, and repeat the stretch. Bring your right elbow under your abdomen and use your body weight to increase the stretch; make sure the direction of the stretch is diagonal. Continue to stretch until the body begins to lengthen. (1 time each side, until accommodation occurs.)

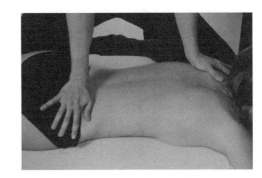

Fig. 10.13

9. Bladder 1 Meridian (bilateral)

Shift position to kneel on one leg. Place your right knee at your client's left trochanter, with your left foot below the left axillary space (fig. 10.14). Your thumbs are resting bilaterally on the Bladder 1 meridian, thumbs pointing cephalically, your fingers spread wide on the dorsum of the rib cage for proprioceptive cueing (fig. 10.15). Apply pressure from the middle of the scapulae (T5) to the middle of the sacrum. Apply moderate pressure perpendicular to the erector spinae cylinder with the ball of the thumb. Be attentive to any reactive points. Be sure you are not thrusting with your thumbs but are instead applying the compressions from your center of gravity. (2 times.)

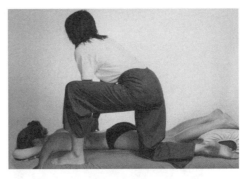

Fig. 10.14

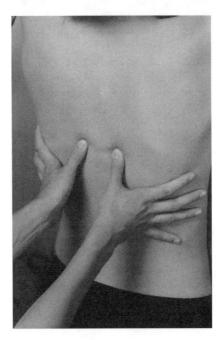

Fig. 10.15

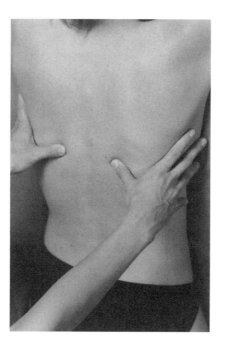

Fig. 10.16

10. Bladder 2 Meridian (bilateral)

Maintaining the same kneeling position, place your thumbs bilaterally on the Bladder 2 meridian, at the lateral margin of the erector spinae muscle mass, thumbs pointing toward each other (fig. 10.16). Apply pressure from the base of the scapulae (T7) to the middle of the gluteals. (Note that the pathway curves around the gluteus medius muscle.) Apply pressure medially at a 45-degree angle, toward the center of the erector spinae cylinder, using moderate tip-of-thumb pressure. (2 times.) **Note:** Avoid the temptation to "push" your thumbs toward each other. Because of the finger position, the thumbs will naturally move toward each other when pressure is applied.

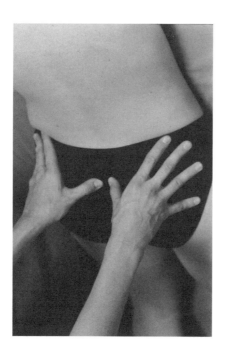

Fig. 10.17

11. Seki Sai Sen—Sacrum

Maintain the same body position, moving to just below your client's pelvis. The tips of your thumbs touch, their pads resting on either side of the spinous processes of the sacrum, the fingers spread wide on the gluteals for proprioceptive cueing (fig. 10.17). Apply pressure on either side of the midline of the sacrum, moving from the sacral base to the sacral apex. Do not press on the coccyx. Use firm ball-of-thumb pressure. (2 times.)

12. Bladder 1 Meridian—Sacrum (bilateral)

Maintaining the same body position, separate your hands so that your thumbs contact the sacral foramina (fig. 10.18). Using firm ball-of-thumb compression, apply perpendicular pressure from the sacral base to the sacral apex. (2 times.)

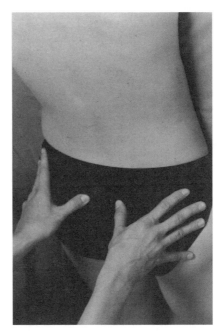

Fig. 10.18

13. Bladder 2 Meridian—Sacrum (bilateral)

Maintaining the same body position, place your thumbs on the lateral margin of the sacrum (fig. 10.19). Apply pressure medially at a 45-degree angle into and under that margin, from the PSIS to the sacral apex. Use firm ball-of-thumb pressure. Avoid the temptation to "push" your thumbs toward each other as noted in step 10. (2 times.)

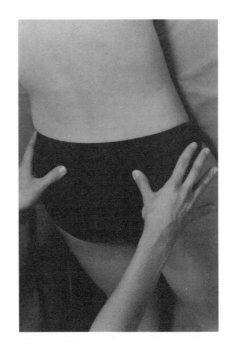

Fig. 10.19

Practice Outline

Back Warm-up

1. Sacral Rocking and Evaluation	Balanced Stance	Until unrestricted
2. Spinal Rocking	Caudal Front Stance	1 time up and down
3. Paraspinal Separation	On table	1 time up and down
4. Rib Mobilization and Thoracic Cross-stretch	On table	1 time up and down
5. Full Cross-stretch	On table	1 time

Reverse instructions and perform steps 2, 3, 4, and 5 on other side.

---

6. Sacral Pumping	On table	3 times each direction
7. Spinal Pump and Stretch	On table	2 times
8. Full Cross-stretch	On table	1 time each side
9. Bladder 1 Meridian (bilateral)	On table	2 times
10. Bladder 2 Meridian (bilateral)	On table	2 times
11. Seki Sai Sen—Sacrum	On table	2 times
12. Bladder 1 Meridian—Sacrum (bilateral)	On table	2 times
13. Bladder 2 Meridian—Sacrum (bilateral)	On table	2 times

CHAPTER 11

TREATMENT OF THE BACK

IN GENERAL, TREAT EACH of the following meridians on the back three times: the first time knocks at the door, the second time asks to enter, and the third time penetrates deeply to the client's comfortable level of tolerance.

1. Seki Sai Sen

Kneel at your client's left side with your left knee at the axilla and the other knee at the hip. Place your thumbs in diamond mudra—tips touching each other at a 45-degree angle—with your fingers spread wide, firmly contacting the far-side erector spinae for proprioceptive cueing (fig. 11.1). Apply pressure in the near-side lamina groove at a 45-degree angle, toward the center of the erector spinae cylinder. Begin at the middle of the scapula (T5) and continue to the middle of the sacrum. Use firm ball-of-thumb pressure. (3 times.) **Note:** Avoid the temptation to "push" your thumbs toward yourself when pressure is applied. Because of the finger position, the thumbs will naturally move toward each other when pressure is applied.

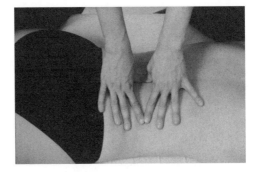

Fig. 11.1

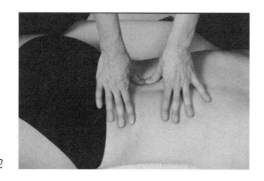

Fig. 11.2

2. Bladder 1 Meridian

Kneeling in the same position, spread your hands moderately apart, with your thumbtips touching at a 180-degree angle (fig. 11.2). Apply perpendicular pressure to the middle of the erector spinae, toward the center of the cylinder. Begin at the middle of the scapula (T5) and work down to the middle of the sacrum. Use firm ball-of-thumb pressure. (3 times.)

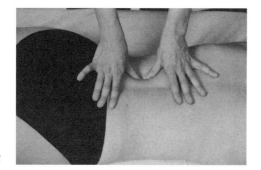

Fig. 11.3

3. Bladder 2 Meridian

Assume a Balanced Stance standing on your client's left side. Direct your line of compression from your center of gravity. With hands parallel and thumbtips touching, the balls of your joined thumbs form one contact point for your compression (fig. 11.3). Apply pressure to the lateral margin of the erector spinae muscle mass at a 45-degree angle toward the spine. Begin at the base of the scapula (T7) and continue to the middle of the gluteus maximus, at the level of the sacral apex, shifting caudally as you reach the ilium. Use firm ball-of-thumb pressure. (3 times.)

4. Gallbladder Meridian

Once again assuming a Balanced Stance, use both thumbs to hook and lift the latissimus dorsi (fig. 11.4). Begin at the axillary border and continue to the common lumbar fascia (fig. 11.5), then curve around the ilium to the anterior superior iliac spine (ASIS) (fig. 11.6). Use broad and gentle thumb pressure on the latissimus dorsi, moderate pressure with thumbs in a T on the common lumbar fascia, and firm thumb-over-thumb pressure on the ilium. (2 times.)

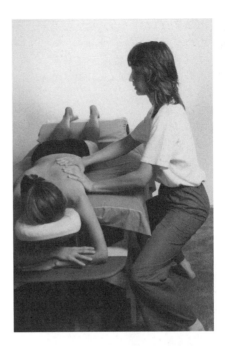

Fig. 11.4

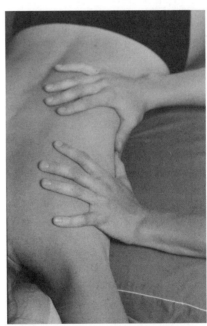

Fig. 11.5

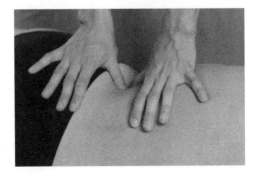

Fig. 11.6

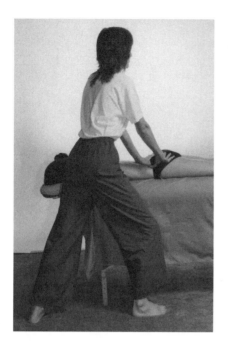

Fig. 11.7

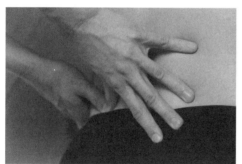

Fig. 11.8

5. Iliac Crest

Standing in a caudal Front Stance, apply thumb-over-thumb pressure along the quadratus lumborum, starting at the transverse process of L5 (fig. 11.7). Compress perpendicular to the lumbar fascia, then hook under the iliac crest and move from the PSIS to the edge of the abdominal obliques (fig. 11.8). Use broad and very firm pressure. (2 times.)

If the lumbar fascia does not yield, stretch your client's leg caudally to open the inguinal region and extend the pelvis flat onto the table, then perform the compression again.

Reverse instructions and perform steps 1 to 5 on the other side.

Practice Outline

The Back

1. Seki Sai Sen	On table	3 times
2. Bladder 1 Meridian	On table	3 times
3. Bladder 2 Meridian	Balanced Stance	3 times
4. Gallbladder Meridian	Balanced Stance	2 times
5. Iliac Crest	Caudal Front Stance	2 times

**Reverse instructions and
perform steps 1 to 5 on the opposite side.**

CHAPTER 12

TREATMENT OF THE HIPS AND BUTTOCKS

THE GROUP OF gluteal muscles is separated into five zones. Pressure is applied at ½-inch intervals along each of the zones. Because of the increased innervation around the anus, pressure in zones 4 and 5 is reduced. Be very mindful not to make inappropriate contact with delicate body areas.

1. Zone 1

Standing at your client's left hip in a caudal Front Stance, fan your fingers and place thumbs in a T (figs. 12.1, 12.2). Begin just lateral to the PSIS and follow the curve of the ilium, ½ inch below the bony crest, to the middle of the tensor fasciae latae. Apply pressure caudally at a 45-degree angle. Use very firm ball-of-thumb pressure. (2 times.)

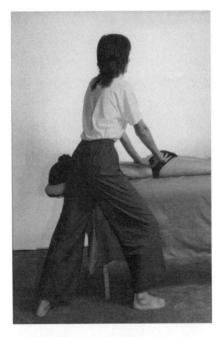

Fig. 12.1

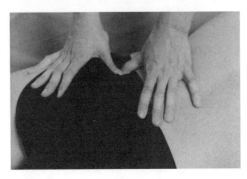

Fig. 12.2

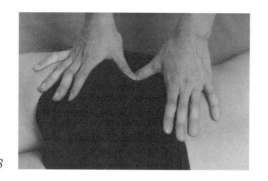

Fig. 12.3

2. Zone 2

Maintaining the same body and hand positions, place thumbs lateral to the second sacral foramen (fig. 12.3). Follow the curve of the ilium, 1½ inches below the bony crest, to the middle of the tensor fasciae latae. Apply perpendicular pressure to the gluteus medius, using broad thumbs and very firm compression. (2 times.)

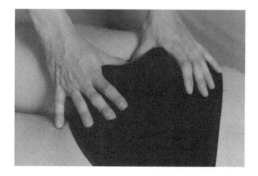

Fig. 12.4

3. Zone 3

Shifting to a Balanced Stance, fan your fingers and place thumbs in a T lateral to the third sacral foramen. Apply pressure straight across the gluteus maximus, to just above the greater trochanter (fig. 12.4). Use broad and firm thumbs to apply perpendicular pressure to the gluteal group. (2 times.)

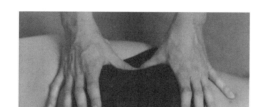

Fig. 12.5

4. Zone 4

Stand at the left hip in a cephalic Back Stance, with hands in the same T position. Beginning ½ inch lateral to the apex of the sacrum, apply pressure in the form of a half moon, curving up to the middle of the greater trochanter (fig. 12.5). Apply pressure perpendicular to the ball of gluteal muscles. Use broad thumbs and moderate pressure. (2 times.)

5. Zone 5

Sinking into a deeper Back Stance, spread the hands wide with thumb over thumb. Begin $\frac{1}{2}$ inch lateral to the edge of the left intergluteal crease and apply pressure cephalically along the inferior gluteal fold. Curve medially to follow the myofascial margin of the gluteus maximus (fig. 12.6). Use broad thumbs and moderate pressure. (2 times.)

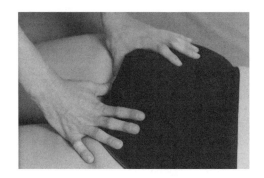

Fig. 12.6

Work on the leg and foot of the same side before reversing instructions and performing steps 1 to 5 on the opposite side.

Practice Outline

Hips and Buttocks

1.	Zone 1	Caudal Front Stance	2 times
2.	Zone 2	Caudal Front Stance	2 times
3.	Zone 3	Balanced Stance	2 times
4.	Zone 4	Cephalic Back Stance	2 times
5.	Zone 5	Deeper Cephalic Back Stance	2 times

Work on the leg and foot of the same side before reversing instructions and performing steps 1 to 5 on the opposite side.

CHAPTER 13

TREATMENT OF THE POSTERIOR LEGS

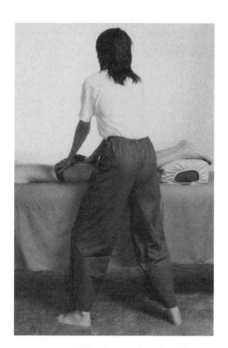

Fig. 13.1

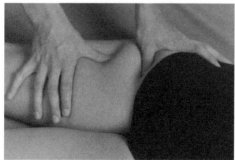

Fig. 13.2

1. Bladder 2 Meridian—Thigh

Standing at your client's left mid-thigh in a closed cephalic Front Stance, use your left hand to support the hip, with the leg in neutral rotation (fig. 13.1). Using the thumb of your right hand, begin at the lateral edge of the inferior buttock crease and apply pressure along the lateral margin of the biceps femoris (fig. 13.2). Continue to the knee crease on the medial margin of the biceps femoris tendon. With your fingers widely spread for support, apply perpendicular pressure to the biceps femoris cylinder. Use moderate ball-of-thumb pressure. (2 times.)

2. Kidney Meridian—Thigh

Standing at mid-calf in a cephalic Back Stance, support the leg at the calf in a slight medial rotation, using your right hand. With the thumb of your left hand apply pressure from the medial margin of the semitendinosus tendon, starting at the popliteal fossa (fig. 13.3). Continue along the semitendinosus to the medial margin of the ischial tuberosity at the subgluteal fold. Apply pressure medially at a 45-degree angle to the hamstring cylinder. Use a very broad and gentle thumb. (2 times.)

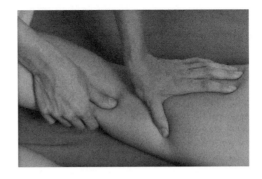

Fig. 13.3

3. Bladder 1 Meridian—Thigh

Stand in an open cephalic Front Stance, hands cupping your client's thigh on either side for support, thumbs in a T. Apply compression beginning just below the ischial tuberosity, in the groove between the hamstrings to the center of the top of the popliteal fossa. Compress perpendicular to the hamstring cylinder, using one broad thumb and the ball of one thumb (fig. 13.4). The pressure is firm. (2 times.)

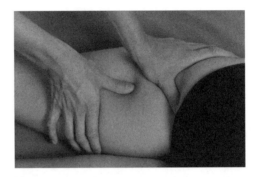

Fig. 13.4

4. Knee Crease

Stand at your client's left mid-calf in a cephalic Front Stance, with your hands surrounding the knee and your thumbtips touching (fig. 13.5). Apply pressure across the knee crease from the center to both edges simultaneously. Then do rainbows (semicircles facing down) on the superior edge of the popliteal fossa, and half-moons (semicircles facing up) on the inferior edge. Apply perpendicular pressure to the popliteal fossa, but only if the leg is bent (the ankle is lifted by a bolster or by your own knee); pressure on the popliteal fossa is contraindicated when the leg is fully extended. Use gentle ball-of-thumb pressure. (2 times.)

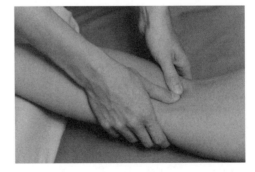

Fig. 13.5

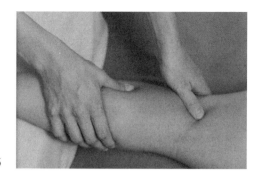

Fig. 13.6

5. Bladder 1 Meridian—Lower Leg

Standing in a cephalic Front Stance at your client's mid-calf, support the leg in neutral rotation with your left hand just above the knee. With the thumb of your right hand begin at the lateral edge of the knee crease and apply pressure along the postero-lateral margin of the gastrocnemius (fig. 13.6). Continue along the groove between the calcaneal tendon and the fibula to the level of the lateral malleolus. Use a broad thumb on the gastrocnemius, and use the ball of your thumb in the groove. (2 times.)

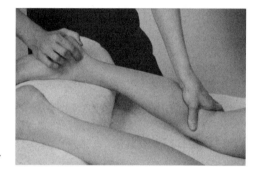

Fig. 13.7

6. Kidney Meridian—Lower Leg

Standing near your client's left foot in a cephalic Back Stance, support your client's leg in a slight medial rotation at the foot with your right hand (fig. 13.7). Begin at the level of the medial malleolus and apply compressions on the groove between the calcaneal tendon and the tibia, and then the postero-medial margin of the gastrocnemius, to the level of the knee crease. Apply pressure directly into the groove, and then use perpendicular pressure on the edge of the gastrocnemius cylinder. Use the ball of your thumb in the groove, and a broad and gentle thumb on the gastrocnemius. (2 times.)

7. Bladder 1 Meridian—Lower Leg

Stand at your client's left mid-leg in a cephalic Front Stance, cupping the leg below the knee crease with your hands, thumbtips touching. Begin at the center of the inferior margin of the popliteal fossa, applying pressure between the heads of the gastrocnemius down through the center of the calcaneal tendon (fig. 13.8). Continue to the calcaneus. Use firm ball-of-thumb pressure. (2 times).

Work on the leg and foot of the same side before reversing instructions and performing steps 1 to 7 on the opposite side.

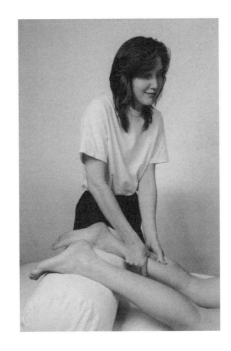

Fig. 13.8

Practice Outline

Posterior Legs

1. Bladder 2 Meridian—Thigh	Cephalic Front Stance	2 times
2. Kidney Meridian—Thigh	Cephalic Back Stance	2 times
3. Bladder 1 Meridian—Thigh	Cephalic Front Stance	2 times
4. Knee Crease	Cephalic Front Stance	2 times
5. Bladder 1 Meridian—Lower Leg	Cephalic Front Stance	2 times
6. Kidney Meridian—Lower Leg	Cephalic Back Stance	2 times
7. Bladder 1 Meridian—Lower Leg	Cephalic Front Stance	2 times

Work on the leg and foot of the same side before reversing instructions and performing steps 1 to 7 on the opposite side.

CHAPTER 14

TREATMENT OF
THE ANKLES AND FEET

FOR TREATMENT OF THE ankles and feet, I alternate between the Front Stance and Back Stance as the particular movement dictates. If you are not using a bolster and your table is wide enough, you can sit on the edge of the table and rest the leg on your thigh to treat the sole of the foot. If you are using a bolster, the position for treating the sole is a Front Stance standing behind the foot.

1. Ankle Stretch

Stand at your client's knee in a cephalic Front Stance. Make sure both of your client's legs are fully extended from the hip with the pelvis flat on the table. Traction them gently toward you, as needed, to open the inguinal groove. With your right hand at the instep and your left hand at the shin, shake the leg back and forth to release muscular holding at the joints. Gently traction the leg as you lower it to the table. Flex the knee and dorsiflex the foot (fig. 14.1). While cupping the ball of the foot with the heel of your right hand and supporting the leg at the heel with your left hand, apply caudal trac-

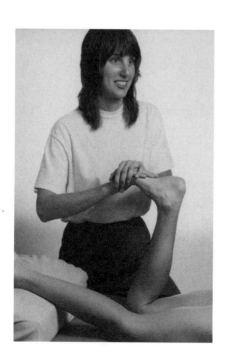

Fig. 14.1

tion on a diagonal vector. Use your body weight directly on the foot to increase and stabilize the stretch. Make sure that you apply your pressure distal to the ball of the foot in order to stretch the plantar fascia. Continue as long as the tendino-fascial complex continues to stretch; hold until the calf muscles stop yielding, then release the leg to the table. (1 time.)

2. Anterior Leg Stretch

Still in a cephalic Front Stance, grasp the left ankle with your left hand. Lift the entire leg, supporting it at the knee with your right hand. Gently traction the thigh to flatten the pelvis. Lower the thigh and flex the knee, left palm on the dorsum of the foot, fingers wrapped over toes (fig. 14.2). Apply pressure cephalically to ensure a complete stretch of the anterior thigh, leg, and dorsum of the foot. Stretch to your client's tolerance, being mindful of any knee problems. Enter into the stretch slowly: if a protective splinting reflex occurs (see page 122), stop the stretch immediately. If the heel presses easily into the buttocks, you can increase the stretch by lifting the knee. (1 time.)

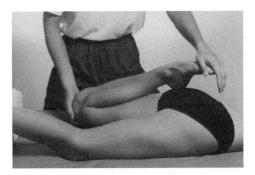

Fig. 14.2

3. Ankle Range-of-Motion

Shift to a cephalic Back Stance. With your client's leg still flexed at the knee, cup the heel with your left hand and grasp the dorsum of the foot at the metatarso-phalangeal junction with your right hand, wrapping your fingers around the toes (fig. 14.3). Lift and slightly traction the ankle, opening the joint. Rotate the foot left and right through its full range of motion while keeping an even stretch on both sides of the joint in every plane of rotation. (3 times in each direction.)

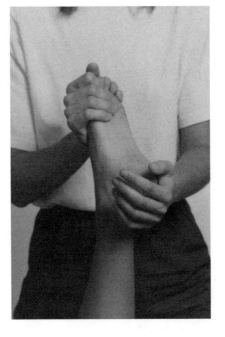

Fig. 14.3

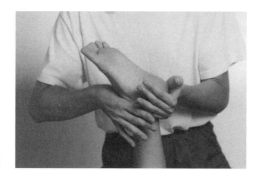

Fig. 14.4

4. Ankle Sawing

Maintaining your posture, cup the calcaneus in your left palm at the metacarpo-phalangeal crease of your fourth metacarpal bone. Your right hand supports the dorsum of the foot at the ankle crease, catching it in the fleshy part of the web between the right thumb and index finger (fig. 14.4). Apply slight traction to the foot to create space in the ankle joint; then rapidly push and pull your hands in opposite directions to produce a loose alternating inversion/eversion movement of the foot. Continue until the ankle releases. (1 time.)

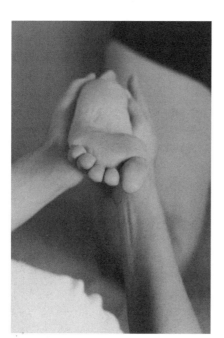

Fig. 14.5

5. Malleolar Infinities

Maintaining the cephalic Back Stance, cup the malleoli in the center of your palms (fig. 14.5). Make rapid alternating circular rotations with both hands until the ankle joint releases. When done correctly, the foot motion will describe a figure eight. (1 time.)

6. Ankle Bracelet

Still in the cephalic Back Stance with your client's leg flexed at the knee, support the medial side of the foot at the toes with your right hand. Apply digital compression with the thumb of your left hand, along the ankle crease, from the medial to the lateral supracalcaneal fossa (fig. 14.6). When you reach the lateral supracalcaneal fossa, pinch the insertion of the Achilles tendon bilaterally with the ball of your thumb and the tip of your index finger. Use moderate pressure. (1 time.)

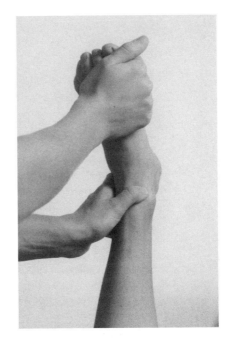

Fig. 14.6

7. Metatarsal Mobilization

Maintaining your posture, grasp the head of the first metatarsal with your right hand, resting your fingers on the sole and your thumb on the dorsum of the foot. Grasp the head of the second metatarsal with your left hand in the same way. Perform an alternating sawing motion to mobilize the interosseous tissues until they move freely. Repeat the movement, sliding your hands laterally on the foot to mobilize the second and third metatarsals, the third and fourth metatarsals (fig. 14.7), and fourth and fifth metatarsals. (1 time.)

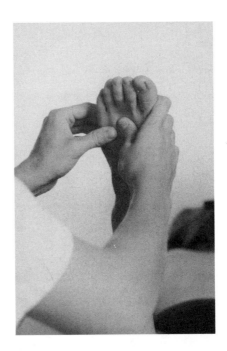

Fig. 14.7

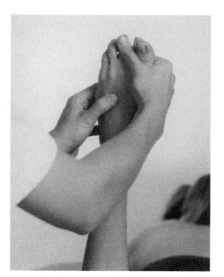

8. Dorsal Zones

Maintain your posture, your client's leg flexed at the knee. Support the ball of the foot with your right hand. With the thumb of your left hand apply digital compressions from the tarsal region to the metatarsal heads, in six zones: on the lateral and medial margins of the foot at the color-change line, and between each pair of metatarsals (fig. 14.8). (2 times.)

Fig. 14.8

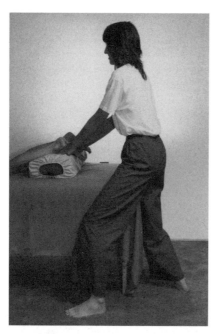

9. Calcaneal Mobilization

Standing at the foot of the table in a Front Stance, cup the sides of the heel between the heels of your hands (fig. 14.9). Moving up and down the edges of the calcaneus, apply alternate circular compressive friction to release the soft tissue (fig. 14.10). (1 time.)

Fig. 14.9

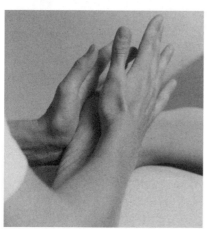

Fig. 14.10

10. Calcaneal Compressions

Supporting the dorsum of your client's foot with the fingers of both hands, apply compressions simultaneously down both edges of the calcaneus with your thumbs (fig. 14.11). Then use both thumbs to compress a line down the center of the heel. (2 times.)

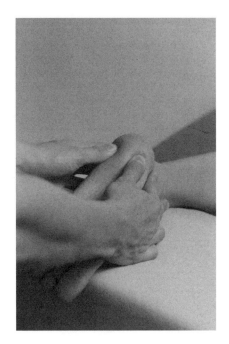

Fig. 14.11

11. Plantar Zones

Support your client's foot with the fingers of both hands cupping the dorsum of the foot. Apply digital pressure with both thumbs, from the inferior calcaneal border to the metatarso-phalangeal joint along five zones: down the midline of the foot, with thumbtips touching (fig. 14.12); halfway out, medially and laterally, between the fourth and fifth and first and second metatarsals simultaneously; and finally down the medial and lateral borders of the foot simultaneously. Gain leverage by pressing against the dorsum of the foot with your fingers. Pressure is applied with the ball of the thumbs, while wrists rotate in a can-opener type of movement. Press deeply, to the client's tolerance level. (2 times.)

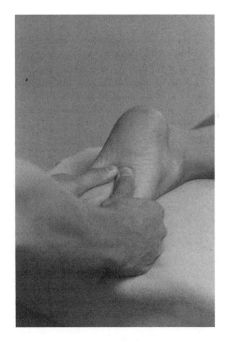

Fig. 14.12

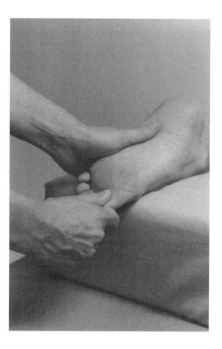

Fig. 14.13

12. Toe Stretch, Roll, and Pinch

Support your client's foot in the middle of the plantar surface with your left hand. Grasp the little toe at the root with your right thumb and index finger, and stretch it by dropping your body weight into a Back Stance. Make a back-and-forth rolling motion while sliding down to the tip of the toe, then pinch the medial and lateral surfaces of the toenail simultaneously. Repeat for the fourth, third, and second toes. Apply traction to the big toe, then rotate it 3 times in each direction (fig. 14.13). Return the foot to the bolster, and cover the plantar surface of the large toe with firm compressions, using the ball of the thumb. (1 time.) **Note:** If the toes make a popping sound while being stretched, hold for a few seconds while the body accommodates to the release before rolling and pinching.

Reverse instructions and perform all steps on the opposite side.

Practice Outline

Ankles and Feet

1. Ankle Stretch	Cephalic Front Stance	1 time
2. Anterior Leg Stretch	Cephalic Front Stance	1 time
3. Ankle Range-of-Motion	Cephalic Back Stance	3 times each direction
4. Ankle Sawing	Cephalic Back Stance	1 time
5. Malleolar Infinities	Cephalic Back Stance	1 time
6. Ankle Bracelet	Cephalic Back Stance	1 time
7. Metatarsal Mobilization	Cephalic Back Stance	1 time
8. Dorsal Zones	Cephalic Back Stance	2 times
9. Calcaneal Mobilization	Front Stance	1 time
10. Calcaneal Compressions	Front Stance	2 times
11. Plantar Zones	Front Stance	2 times
12. Toe Stretch, Roll, and Pinch	Front Stance	1 time

Reverse instructions and perform all steps on the opposite side.

TREATMENT OF THE SCAPULAE AND UPPER ARMS

1. Infrascapular Margin

Move to stand at the left mid-thorax in a cephalic Front Stance. Extend, medially rotate, and adduct your client's arm, placing the wrist on the small of the back. (If this position is painful for your client, leave the arm alongside the body but bring the hand up toward the shoulder, abducting the elbow.) Slide your left palm flat under the deltoid muscle and lightly bounce the shoulder to release the rhomboids, being careful not to use poking pressure on the pecto-deltoid region. With your right hand apply a sawing motion with the radial edge of your index finger along the infrascapular region from the inferior medial angle of the scapula at T7 to the point where the trapezius overlies the scapula at T3 (fig. 15.1). Work as deeply under the scapula as your client's tolerance will allow. (2 times.)

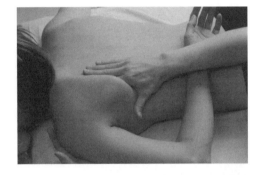

Fig. 15.1

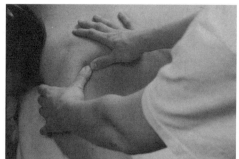

Fig. 15.2

2. Small Intestine Meridian—Infraspinatus

Stand facing your client's shoulder in a cephalic Front Stance. Draw the arm away from the body to a 90-degree angle. Spread your fingers wide, thumbtips touching (fig. 15.2). Work from the medial edge of the scapula to the axillary margin along three lines on the infraspinatus: compress the superior margin of the muscle, just below the scapular spine, at a 45-degree angle caudally; next compress across the middle of the muscle, applying perpendicular pressure; finally, compress along the inferior margin, just above the lateral groove (the groove medial to the insertion of the teres major and minor muscles) at a 45-degree angle cephalically. All compressions are toward the center of the infraspinatus cylinder. Use the ball of your thumbs, applying firm pressure. (2 times.)

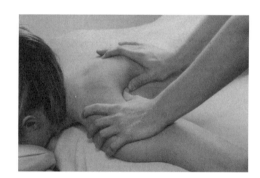

Fig. 15.3

3. Teres Major and Minor

Move one step down and shift to a deep cephalic Front Stance. Spread your fingers wide and hook your thumbs under the lateral margin of the scapula (fig. 15.3). Jostle the teres muscles to loosen them, then work the teres group from the inferior angle to the axilla. Use broad thumbs and firm pressure. Finish by applying firm pressure into the axillary crease with a very broad thumb. (2 times.)

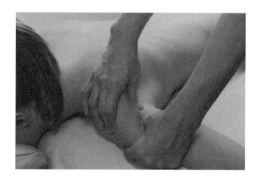

Fig. 15.4

4. Medial and Posterior Deltoids

Shift to an open cephalic Front Stance. Jostle the medial and posterior heads of the deltoid muscle and the entire triceps. Using your thumbs and the palmar surface of your fingers, alternately pluck the tissue over the course of the medial and posterior heads of the deltoid, from distal to proximal (fig. 15.4). Use firm pressure. (2 times.)

5. Large Intestine, Triple Heater, and Small Intestine Meridians—Triceps

With your client's arm still open at a 90-degree angle, shift to a more open cephalic Front Stance. Beginning just above the elbow, alternately pluck the entire triceps muscle, to the deltoid (fig. 15.5). (2 times.)

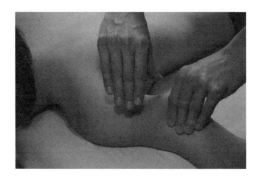

Fig. 15.5

Reverse instructions and perform all steps on the opposite side.

Practice Outline

Scapulae and Upper Arms

1. Infrascapular Margin	Cephalic Front Stance	2 times
2. Small Intestine Meridian—Infraspinatus	Cephalic Front Stance	2 times
3. Teres Major and Minor	Deep Cephalic Front Stance	2 times
4. Medial and Posterior Deltoids	Cephalic Front Stance	2 times
5. Large Intestine, Triple Heater, and Small Intestine Meridians—Triceps	Open Cephalic Front Stance	2 times

Reverse instructions and perform all steps on the opposite side.

CHAPTER 16

TREATMENT OF THE UPPER BACK

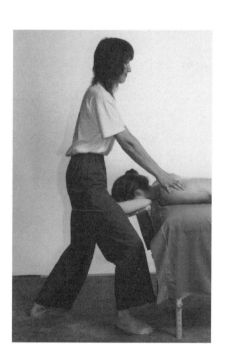

Fig. 16.1

1. Scapular Infinities

Place your client's arms by his sides. Stand at the head of the table in a Front Stance (fig. 16.1). Hook the heels of your palms over the spines of the scapulae (fig. 16.2). Alternately push the scapulae, moving them in a figure-eight pattern—each scapula representing half of the figure eight—to release the circumscapular musculature. Continue until the tissues release and the scapulae move freely.

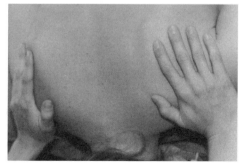

Fig. 16.2

2. Seki Sai Sen (bilateral)

Maintaining the same posture, spread your fingers wide for proprioceptive cueing. Using the balls of your thumbs, apply bilateral pressure into the lamina groove from T5 to T1 (fig. 16.3). Being careful not to press on the spinous processes, first apply entry-level pressure perpendicularly into the groove lateral to the spinous processes. In the second pass, apply firm lateral pressure into the cylinder of the erector spinae. (2 times.)

3. Bladder 1 Meridian—Medial Trapezius (bilateral)

Maintaining the same posture, use the balls of your thumbs to apply bilateral pressure perpendicularly into the middle of the erector spinae cylinder, from T5 to T1 (fig. 16.4). When you reach T1, lower your stance and shift the direction of your pressure so it is perpendicular to the medial trapezius along the midline (coronal axis) (fig. 16.5); work out to the acromion process. Use firm pressure. (2 times.)

Note: Be mindful that the coracoid process of the scapula is just medial to the acupoint Gb21. If it feels like you are pressing on a bone, you probably are.

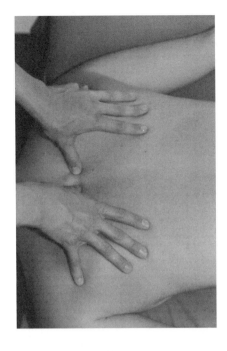

Fig. 16.3

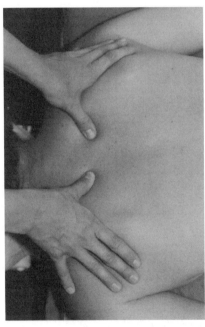

Fig. 16.4

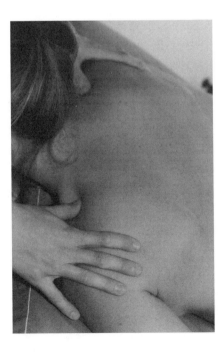

Fig. 16.5

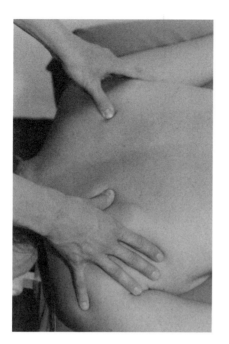

Fig. 16.6

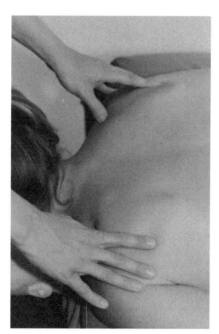

Fig. 16.7

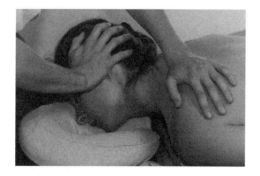

Fig. 16.8

4. Bladder 2 Meridian— Supraspinous Fossa (bilateral)

Maintaining the same posture, apply bilateral pressure with the tips of your thumbs to the lateral edge of the erector spinae cylinder from T7 to T3, directing your pressure medially 45 degrees into the cylinder (fig. 16.6). At T3, shift your direction to work out to the end of the scapular spine, applying firm ball-of-thumb pressure 45 degrees caudal into the supraspinous fossae (fig. 16.7). (2 times.)

5. Cervico-thoracic Mobilization

Standing in a lateral Front Stance in the direction opposite to the way you turn your client's head, rotate your client's head so the right side of the face is on the table or face cradle. Fully extend the neck. Cup your client's left temporo-parietal region with your right hand, the heel of the palm resting on the zygoma; cross your left hand over your right, cupping the medial edge of the scapular spine with the heel of your hand (fig. 16.8). Alternate pressure between the skull and scapula 4 or 5 times, until movement through the cervico-thoracic spine occurs freely. Do not hold this position longer than necessary to perform the stretch. (If you observe protective splinting [see page 122] either when you rotate the neck or when you begin the distractive traction, be very careful. Resistance that does not immediately abate indicates a vertebral subluxation; in this situation, extended range-of-movement stretches will be painful to the client.) Reverse directions to treat the opposite side. When finished, gently direct your client's head to face down in the face cradle. (1 time each side.)

6. Seki Sai Sen (unilateral)

Standing in a Front Stance slightly to the right of the client's midline, fan your fingers and place thumb over thumb at T5. Apply entry-level pressure perpendicularly into the lamina groove alongside the spinous processes, working up to T1 (fig. 16.9). (Be careful not to press on the spinous processes.) The second time apply firm and steady pressure at 45 degrees lateral into the erector spinae cylinder, pressing deep to the client's tolerance. (2 times.)

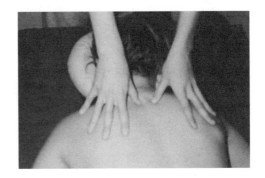

Fig. 16.9

7. Bladder 1 Meridian—Medial Trapezius

Maintaining the same body and hand positions, adjust your stance in small increments to align your center of gravity with the area being treated. Apply perpendicular pressure into the erector spinae cylinder from T5 to T1 (fig. 16.10). Then lower your stance and shift your pressure so it is perpendicular to the medial head of the trapezius, along the midline; work out to the acromion process (fig. 16.11). Pressure is very firm. (2 times.) **Note:** Be mindful that the coracoid process of the scapula is just medial to the acupoint Gb21. If it feels like you are pressing on a bone, you probably are.

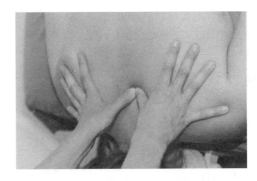

Fig. 16.10

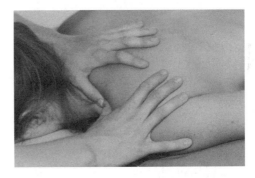

Fig. 16.11

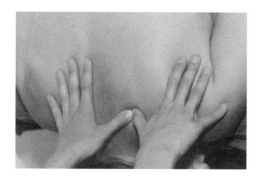

Fig. 16.12

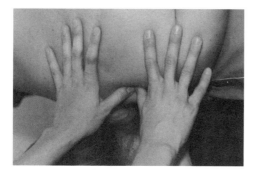

Fig. 16.13

8. Bladder 2 Meridian— Supraspinous Fossa

Maintaining the same body and hand positions, apply pressure to the lateral edge of the erector spinae from T7 to T3 (fig. 16.12). First press medially at a 45-degree angle into the erector spinae, then shift your pressure to 45 degrees caudal, into the supraspinous fossa. Work out to the end of the scapular spine (fig. 16.13). Pressure is very firm and steady. (2 times.)

Reverse instructions for steps 6, 7, and 8 and perform on the opposite side.

9. Scapular Infinities

To finish treatment of the upper back, repeat Scapular Infinities. See instructions on page 154.

Practice Outline

Upper Back

1. Scapular Infinities	Front Stance at head of table	Until unrestricted
2. Seki Sai Sen (bilateral)	Front Stance at head of table	2 times
3. Bladder 1 Meridian— Medial Trapezius (bilateral)	Front Stance at head of table	2 times
4. Bladder 2 Meridian— Supraspinous Fossa (bilateral)	Front Stance at head of table	2 times
5. Cervico-thoracic Mobilization	Lateral Front Stance	1 time each side
6. Seki Sai Sen (unilateral)	Front Stance at head of table	2 times
7. Bladder 1 Meridian— Medial Trapezius (unilateral)	Front Stance shifting in small increments	2 times
8. Bladder 2 Meridian— Supraspinous Fossa (unilateral)	Front Stance shifting in small increments	2 times

Reverse instructions for steps 6, 7, and 8 and perform on the opposite side.

9. Scapular Infinities	Front Stance at head of table	

CHAPTER 17

TREATMENT OF THE NECK

Work on the neck is done on one side at a time, treating first the posterior pathways and then the anterior pathways, followed by extended range-of-motion stretching.

Although all of the meridians on the neck are Yang, treatment is applied in both directions. Those meridians beginning on the face and ending at the feet are treated from the occiput to the cervico-thoracic juncture; those beginning at the hand and ending on the face are treated from the base of the neck to the occiput. Note also that the Stomach Meridian is unique among the Yang meridians in having its trajectory along the ventral surface of the body.

At this point in the BodyWork Shiatsu treatment the client turns supine, lying so that the top of the head is 2 inches below the top of your table. Seat yourself at the head of the table, at such a height that your table is level with your chest and you can extend your arms straight out in front of you as you work (fig. 17.1). An adjustable stool is a great asset.

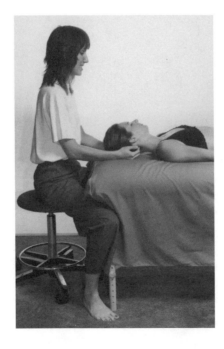

Fig. 17.1

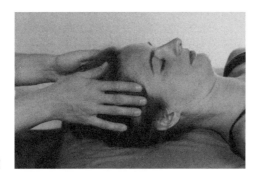

Fig. 17.2

1. Cranial Rocking

Gently grasp the temporal region of the cranium with the fingertips of both hands (fig. 17.2). Rock the head back and forth gently to release residual muscular contraction.

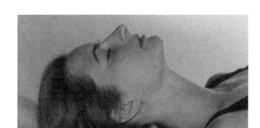

Fig. 17.3

2. Suboccipital Release

Placing your fingertips evenly along the cranial base, slowly and gradually lift your client's head by extending your fingers (fig. 17.3). Maintain pad-of-fingertip contact with the inferior edge of the occiput. The force of the compression is generated entirely by the weight of the client's head. Carefully monitor release of the suboccipital musculature; as the suboccipital triangle opens and your fingertips begin to penetrate the superficial musculature, slowly add a lateral vector to your compression. This serves to widen the base of the occiput and release the trapezius and suboccipital insertions.

As the suboccipital musculature releases and your fingertips contact the second cervical vertebra (the axis), the chin will gradually rise. If the neck splints, encourage your client to allow the back of his or her head to fall into your palms. Hold until a release occurs, or until your hands become too tired to continue.

3. Seki Sai Sen

Supporting the cranium with your left hand at the temporo-occipital prominence, rotate the face to the left. Working with your first three fingers but focusing the compression from your middle finger, apply perpendicular entry-level pressure into the lamina groove of the vertebrae on the right side, from the base of the occiput to the cervico-thoracic junction (fig. 17.4). Then shift the pressure laterally, applying small circular compressions to the superior head of the trapezius. (3 times.)

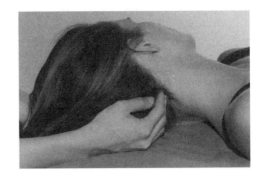

Fig. 17.4

4. Bladder 1 Meridian

Maintaining your support of the cranium, shift your fingers to the latero-posterior margin of the upper trapezius (fig. 17.5). Apply pressure in small circular frictions on the right side from the occiput to the base of the neck. (3 times.)

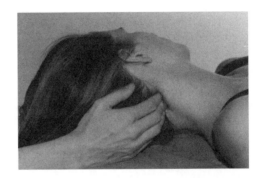

Fig. 17.5

5. Gallbladder Meridian

Still supporting the cranium, shift your fingers slightly to the lateral margin of the upper trapezius, level with the mastoid process (fig. 17.6). Apply pressure in small circular frictions from the base of the occiput to the base of the neck. The posterior aspect of the transverse processes are your deep landmark. (3 times.)

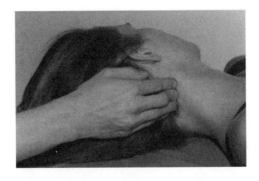

Fig. 17.6

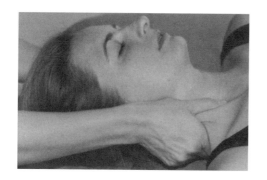

Fig. 17.7

6. Stomach Meridian

Gently guide the cranium back to neutral. Maintaining your support of the cranium, apply gentle, lateral pressure with the ball of your slightly bent thumb along the medial aspect of the sternocleidomastoid, from the insertion at the mastoid process to its origin at the clavicle (fig. 17.7).

Caution: To avoid any irritation to the trachea, pressure must be applied on a sharp lateral diagonal by bending the distal phalanx of your thumb. Press very gently in the area halfway down the neck, so as not to compress the thyroid and parathyroid glands. (2 times.)

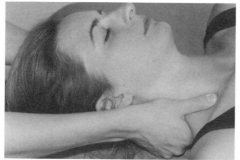
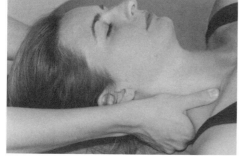

Fig. 17.8

7. Large Intestine Meridian

Continuing to support the cranium, apply gentle perpendicular pressure with the ball of your thumb from the clavicle along the lateral margin of the sternocleidomastoid to the occiput (fig. 17.8). Be careful not to press directly on the mastoid process. (2 times.)

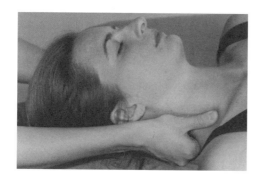

Fig. 17.9

8. Small Intestine Meridian

Continuing to support the cranium, apply firm perpendicular pressure to the lateral aspect of the posterior scalene with the ball of your thumb from the clavicle to the occiput (fig. 17.9). The anterior aspect of the transverse processes are your deep landmarks. (2 times.) **Note:** Pressure on the brachial plexus may cause a reflex radiation down the arm. If this happens, lighten your pressure and continue.

Reverse instructions for steps 3 to 8 and perform on the opposite side.

EXTENDED RANGE-OF-MOTION STRETCHING

Extended range-of-motion stretching exercises, such as those described in steps 9–13, help greatly in developing the therapist's proprioceptive awareness. Range-of-motion stretching allows you to reset the client's muscle resting-length pattern held in his or her neurology. To perform these stretches successfully, a therapist must be familiar with the rate and timing of myofascial lengthening within his or her own body. This only comes from the practice of appropriate stretching techniques.* In extended range-of-motion stretching the therapist must maintain a constant, subtle state of reciprocal communication with the client's body. This involves both proprioceiving the incremental releases of the myofascial tissues and feeding back the appropriate encouragement to the client's neuromusculature. The action must be slow and gentle, yet firm enough to overcome the unconscious restrictive contractures patterned in the client's nervous system.

Do not overstretch the neck, as this will only produce a painful rebound contraction later. Subluxed, or partially dislocated, vertebrae will create a painful pinching sensation when stretched; if this occurs, as evidenced by verbal exclamations or protective splinting (see page 122), stop the stretch.

Stretched joints should be returned to an anatomically neutral position by the therapist. If your client actively assists in the return movement, the released myofascial tissues will contract again, thereby defeating the potential for neuromuscular reeducation. Ask that the client be totally passive and allow you to complete the return movement. Perform the return movements very slowly so as to allow the nervous system time to integrate the new information. Pause briefly between stretches for the same reason. Distractive oscillation (see page 123) should be performed after each return.

---

* Such stretching techniques include any of the nonballistic, volitional movements that focus on the slow and conscious release of tissue tension, with a gradual, incremental lengthening of the affected muscles. A practice such as hatha yoga or Hanna Somatics, which includes a conscious review and release of residual tension throughout the body, is also very helpful.

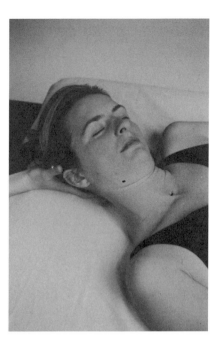

Fig. 17.10

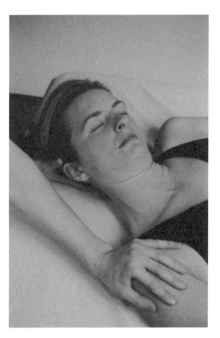

Fig. 17.11

9. Lateral Stretch

Support the cranium at the parietal prominence with your right hand (fig. 17.10). Place the flat of your left palm on the acromion process of the right shoulder (fig. 17.11). Actively restraining the shoulder, traction your client's neck to the left, to the full limit of its range of motion. Create a biased vector of stretch by firmly anchoring the shoulder while stretching the neck. The vector of stretch is superior and lateral, with the intent of lengthening the entire cervical region, not just the lateral aspect. Pressure must be firm and steady. Pay close attention to proprioceptive feedback; never force the stretch or stretch past your client's range of motion. After advising your client to be completely passive, very slowly return the head to an anatomically neutral position.

Reverse the instructions and perform the stretch on the opposite side.

---

10. Anterior Stretch

Lift your client's head with both hands, to the limit of anterior flexion. Cup the occipital prominences in the palms of your hands, resting your elbows on the table for support (fig. 17.12, 17.13). The cranium is antero-flexed by a rotation from your wrists; the vector of stretch is upward and outward rather than simply forward. Maintain a gentle but constant traction throughout the stretch. After requesting your client to remain passive, fully support the head and slowly return it to the table (fig. 17.14).

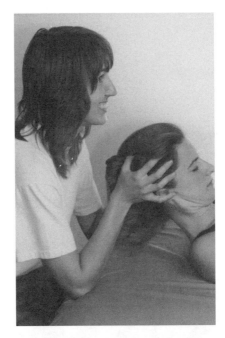

Fig. 17.12

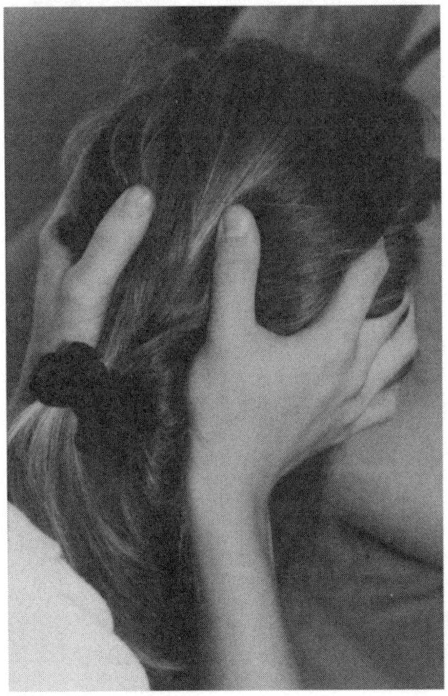

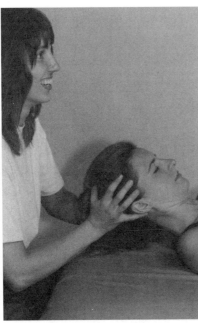

Fig. 17.13

Fig. 17.14

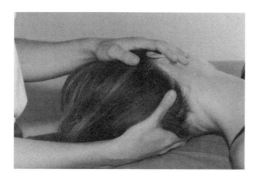

Fig. 17.15

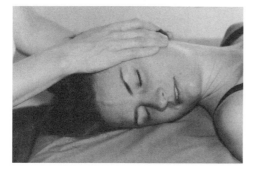

Fig. 17.16

11. Lateral Rotation

Laterally rotate your client's head to the left, with your right hand cupping the cranium at the left parietal prominence and your left hand resting on the right cheek over the zygomatic process (fig. 17.15). Slightly extend and rotate the neck to the limit of its lateral range of motion. Then gently rotate the head between your hands: 70 percent of the rotational force is applied with your left hand, 30 percent with your right (fig. 17.16). Gently oscillate the cranium in a supero-inferior direction to defeat any protective splinting (see page 122). Do not overstretch. Remind your client to be completely passive, and very slowly return the head to an anatomically neutral position.

Reverse the instructions and perform the stretch on the opposite side.

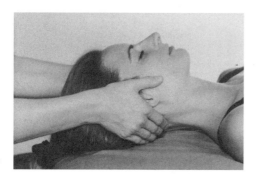

Fig. 17.17

12. Manual Traction

Gently oscillate your client's head several times to release any residual splinting. Grasp the cranium with both hands: place the last three fingers at the base of the occiput with the thumb resting on the mandibular angle, its distal phalanx hooked under the mandibular notch (fig. 17.17). Bracing your knees against the table, very slowly apply traction to the limit of cervical extension, using your body weight rather than your arm strength to effect the traction. Maintain the cephalic traction until post-splinting release occurs (10 to 15 seconds). Then slowly release your body weight while maintaining cephalic traction with your arm, until accommodation occurs once again (5 to 10 seconds). If necessary, remind your client to release the cervical musculature. Eighty to 90 percent of the tractioning force is generated by your fingers under the occiput; your thumb under the mandible provides a stabilizing and supporting influence. Subluxed vertebrae will cause protective splinting of the cervical musculature (see page 122) and can prevent the successful application of traction. If you suspect a subluxed vertebra(e), do not perform this stretch.

13. Cranial Rocking

Finish extended range-of-motion stretching with cranial rocking as described on page 160.

Practice Outline

The Neck

All techniques are performed with the practitioner seated at the head of the table.

1. Cranial Rocking		
2. Suboccipital Release		
3. Seki Sai Sen	Superior to inferior	3 times
4. Bladder 1 Meridian	Superior to inferior	3 times
5. Gallbladder Meridian	Superior to inferior	3 times
6. Stomach Meridian	Superior to inferior	2 times
7. Large Intestine Meridian	Inferior to superior	2 times
8. Small Intestine Meridian	Inferior to superior	2 times

Repeat steps 3 through 8 on the opposite side.

---

9. Lateral Stretch	Both sides
10. Anterior Stretch	
11. Lateral Rotation	Both sides
12. Manual Traction	
13. Cranial Rocking	

TREATMENT OF THE FACE

A S W H E N T R E A T I N G the neck, the practitioner is seated at the head of the table in
order to treat the face.

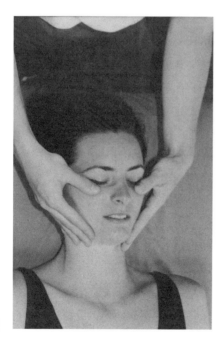

Fig. 18.1

1. Infraorbital Plane

Beginning alongside the nose, apply bilateral pressure to the infraorbital fossa, from the inner to the
outer corners of the eye, with gentle ball-of-thumb
pressure (fig. 18.1). Be careful not to close off the
nostrils. Apply pressure at a 45-degree angle,
obliquely inferior. (2 times.)

2. Zygomatic Process

Beginning alongside the nostrils, apply perpendicular pressure along the zygomatic arch to just beyond the suture with the temporal process (fig. 18.2). Use firm ball-of-thumb pressure. Be careful not to close off the nostrils. (2 times.)

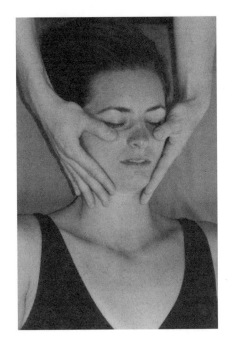

Fig. 18.2

3. Infrazygomatic Fossa

Beginning lateral to the nostrils, hook your thumb under and into the tissues beneath the zygomatic process (fig. 18.3). Work laterally to just beyond the suture with the temporal process. Apply moderate pressure using the tips of your thumbs. Be careful not to close off the nostrils. (2 times.)

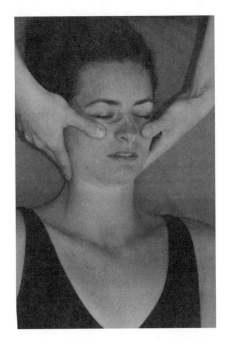

Fig. 18.3

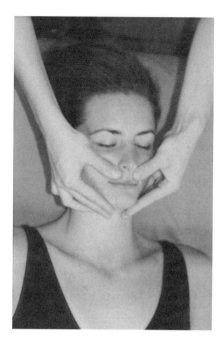

Fig. 18.4

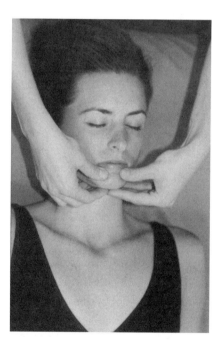

Fig. 18.5

4. Mouth

Begin in the center of the mentolabial groove of the upper lip, with your thumbtips touching. Use the broad balls of your thumbs to press up and out (fig. 18.4). Apply pressure every ½ inch, following the curve of the lip to the corners. The direction of pressure is always lateral and away from the mouth. Once at the outer corners, skip to the center line of the lower lip, ½ inch below the lip itself, and follow the curve out to the corners (fig. 18.5). Give special attention to the points just lateral to the edges of the mouth. This is a tissue-spreading technique; it does not involve actual stretching of the lip membrane. (2 times.)

Caution: Be especially gentle when treating clients with dry lips so that your compressions do not crack the lips. You must lighten your pressure when clients wearing dentures automatically tighten their lips for protection.

5. Mandible

Starting in the central groove of the mandible, bring your thumbs and first two fingers into a pinching position (kitty paws) (fig. 18.6). Compress the flesh over the mandible against the bone every ½ inch out to the mandibular angle. Apply pressure along the supero-lateral margin of the mandible at a 45-degree angle. (2 times.)

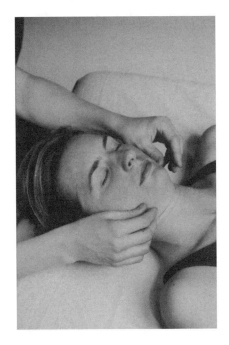

Fig. 18.6

6. Eye Zones

Carefully place the heels of your palms on the forehead, resting your distal phalanges on the zygomatic arch for proprioceptive cueing to determine the right degree of support before applying compression to the eyes (fig. 18.7). Press gently on the closed eyelids with the proximal phalanx of your thumbs over three zones, medial to lateral. Be careful not to press down with the balls of your thumbs or to apply heavy pressure to the eyelids in any way. This compression should not be done on a client wearing contact lenses. (2 times.)

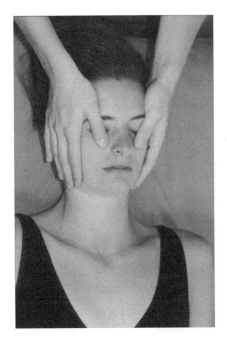

Fig. 18.7

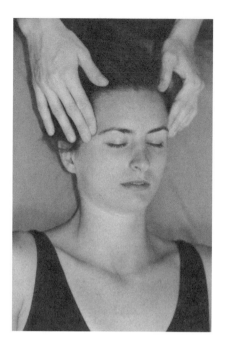

Fig. 18.8

7. Temple Points

Place your index fingers, reinforced by your middle fingers, on the temple points ½ inch lateral to the orbit of the eye in the sphenoid fossa (fig. 18.8). Perform small circular frictions over the points. Be gentle at first, gradually increasing your pressure as the tissues soften and release. (2 times.)

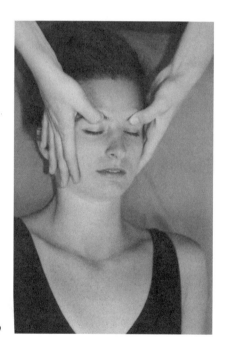

Fig. 18.9

8. Eyebrows

Place the heels of your palms on your client's forehead for proprioceptive cueing to determine the right degree of support before applying compression to the eyebrows. Begin infero-medial to the eyebrows and work supero-laterally, through the grooves that pass through the middle of the eyebrows. Begin with the balls of thumbs bent, straightening them to conform to the angle of the frontal bone (fig. 18.9). Be very careful not to press into the eyeballs. (2 times.)

9. Forehead Zones

Begin with your thumbtips touching, just above the centerline of the eyebrows. Compress three zones laterally: just above the eyebrows, in the middle of the forehead, and on the natural hairline (fig. 18.10). Continue to the temporoparietal suture, about 1 inch into the temporal fossa. Pressure on the frontal bones can be very heavy, but it must be light on the temporal fossae. **Note:** The natural hairline may be found on mature males by asking them to raise their eyebrows. The natural hairline is at the junction of the frontalis muscle and the galea aponeurotica, and will be obvious. (2 times.)

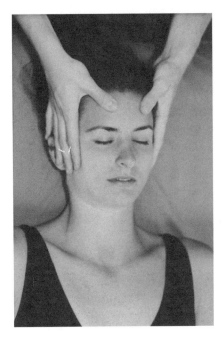

Fig. 18.10

Practice Outline

The Face

All techniques are performed with the practitioner seated at the head of the table.

1. Infraorbital Plane	2 times
2. Zygomatic Process	2 times
3. Infrazygomatic Fossa	2 times
4. Mouth	2 times
5. Mandible	2 times
6. Eye Zones	2 times
7. Temple Points	2 times
8. Eyebrows	2 times
9. Forehead Zones	2 times

CHAPTER 19

TREATMENT OF THE HEAD

T HE TREATMENT OF the head is performed with the practitioner seated at the head of the table.

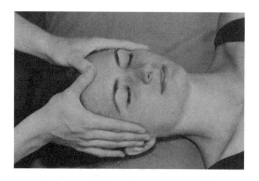

Fig. 19.1

1. Governor Vessel

Begin at GV20, in the slight depression at the top of the head that is even with the superior border of the external ear (fig. 19.1). Apply thumb-over-thumb pressure along the midsagittal line to the glabela, the hollow just superior to the meeting of the eyebrow ridges. Pressure should be moderate on the parietal suture and very firm on the frontal bone. (2 times.)

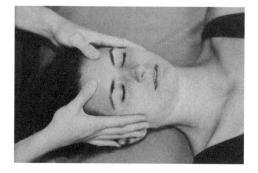

Fig. 19.2

2. Bladder Meridian

Beginning at the medial corners of the eyebrows, apply compressions up the frontal bone, gradually widening the distance between your thumbs until they are ½ inch on either side of midsagittal line at the natural hairline (fig. 19.2). Then work directly back, through the parietal bones, to the apex of the head. Use heavy pressure on the frontal bone and moderate pressure on the parietal bones. (2 times.)

3. First Gallbladder Line

Starting at the lateral edge of the eyebrows, apply pressure along the temporalis muscle insertions. Follow the superior parietal ridges to the parietal eminences (fig. 19.3). Use the lateral edge of your thumbs with moderate pressure. (2 times.)

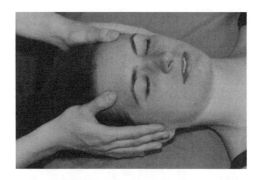

Fig. 19.3

4. Second Gallbladder Line

Using the pads of your first three fingers, apply pressure in a zigzag pattern (fig. 19.4). Follow a curved course through the temporal fossa, from the anterior hairline (about three inches above the outer edge of the ears) to the occipital bone. The aim of this movement is to mobilize the tissue over the temporal fossae; pressure should be light and smooth. (2 times.)

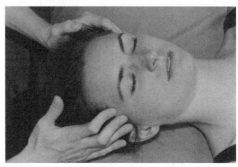

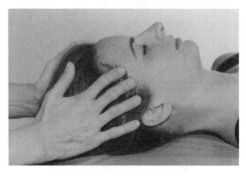

Fig. 19.4

5. Triple Heater Line

Starting just above the edge of the ears, use your middle two fingertips to apply pressure in a zigzag pattern moving bilaterally from above the zygomatic arch to the root of the mastoid process, following the outer contour of the external auditory meatus (figs. 19.5, 19.6, 19.7). (2 times.)

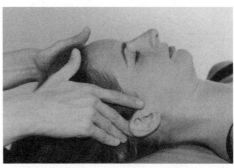

Fig. 19.5

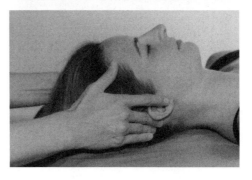

Fig. 19.6

Fig. 19.7

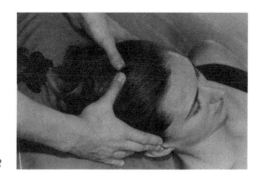

Fig. 19.8

6. First Horizontal Line

Start with your thumbtips touching at the mid-sagittal line, even with the front of the ears (fig. 19.8). Apply bilateral compressions along the coronal suture to the squamosal suture. Use moderate ball-of-thumb pressure on the parietal bones, lightening your pressure as you reach the temporal fossae. (2 times.)

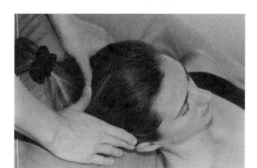

Fig. 19.9

7. Second Horizontal Line

Start with thumbtips touching at the midsagittal line, even with the tip of the ears (fig. 19.9). Apply bilateral compressions along the lambdoidal suture to the squamosal suture. Use moderate ball-of-thumb pressure on the parietal bones, lightening your pressure as you reach the temporal fossae. (2 times.)

Practice Outline

The Head

All techniques are performed with the practitioner seated at the head of the table.

1. Governor Vessel	2 times
2. Bladder Meridian	2 times
3. First Gallbladder Line	2 times
4. Second Gallbladder Line	2 times
5. Triple Heater Line	2 times
6. First Horizontal Line	2 times
7. Second Horizontal Line	2 times

TREATMENT OF THE ABDOMEN

WHEN TREATING the abdomen, the client lies supine with arms at the sides, knees flexed and feet drawn up toward the pelvis to release the abdominal recti. The use of an eight- or nine-inch bolster under the knees is very effective. It is best that your client not have eaten within two hours prior to treatment. If treatment must be given within two hours after eating, omit step 7 (Stomach Sawing).

1. Lumbar Oscillation

Standing in a cephalic Front Stance on the client's left side, just superior to the pelvis, hold your client at the waist (fig. 20.1). Place the medial surface of your index fingers on the lateral margin of the torso against either side of the flank (between the twelfth rib and the ilium), thumbs resting on the torso (fig 20.2). Begin an alternate rocking movement to mobilize the large intestine and lumbar region. Continue until the movement becomes unrestricted—the pelvis and the torso will begin to move as separate segments between your hands.

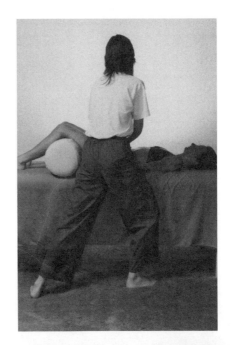

Fig. 20.1

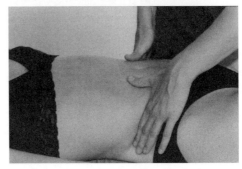

Fig. 20.2

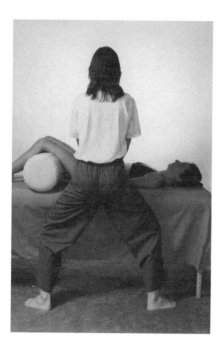

Fig. 20.3

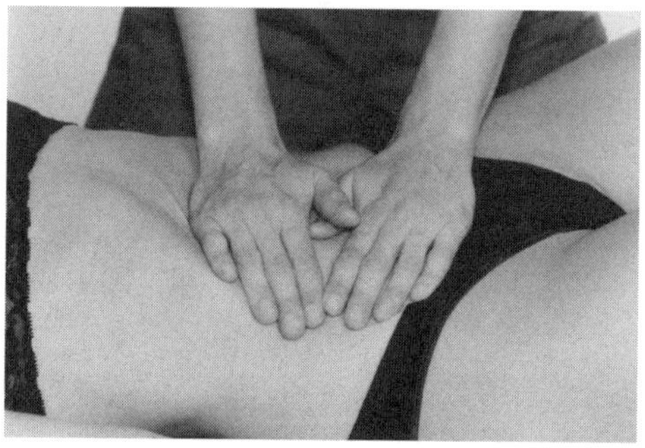

Fig. 20.4

2. Abdominal Rocking

Shifting to a wide Balanced Stance, place your palms flat across the abdominal surface, thumbs touching along their length (figs. 20.3, 20.4). Be careful not to apply pressure on either the pubic bone or the costal border. Perform a wavelike, horizontal figure-eight rocking motion to mobilize the abdominal contents. Press gently down with the heels of the hands, then push forward, rolling the palms across the abdomen. Complete the movement by pressing down on the opposite side with the fingers, then pull your hands back toward you while rolling your palms back across the abdomen. Pressure must be even throughout the range of movement. (10 to 15 times.)

3. Large Intestine

Maintaining the same position, place the pads of the first three fingers of the left hand over the ileo-cecal valve, midway between the ASIS and the navel on the right side. The fingers of the right hand lie on top of the left for support (fig. 20.5). Pressure is applied with the right hand, while the fingertips of the left hand sense the tonus of the tissues being treated. Perform circular friction over the ascending, transverse, descending, and sigmoid colon, moving about 1 inch between compressions (figs. 20.6, 20.7, 20.8). Begin with easy pressure and increase gradually each time, to comfortable client tolerance. (3 times.)

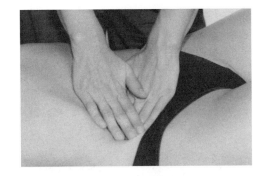

Fig. 20.5

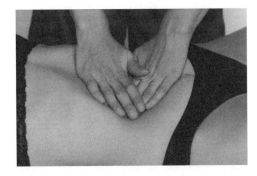

Fig. 20.6

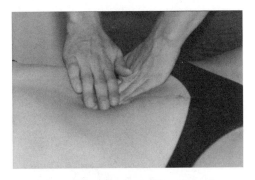

Fig. 20.7

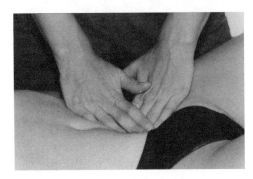

Fig. 20.8

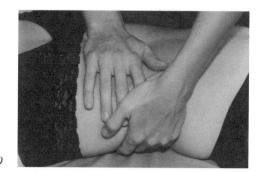

Fig. 20.9

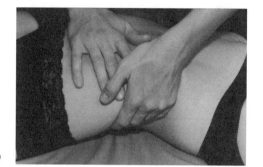

Fig. 20.10

4. Liver/Rib Mobilization

Shift to a cephalic Front Stance. Slip your left hand under the lower right rib cage, placing your right hand on the top of the rib cage (fig. 20.9). Alternately pump with one hand and then the other to mobilize the rib cage (fig. 20.10). Continue until the ribs move freely.

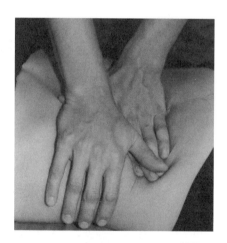

Fig. 20.11

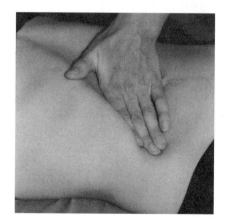

Fig. 20.12

5. Liver Sawing

Maintaining the same stance, fan the fingers of your right hand to firmly support the right anterior ribs. Then with the thenar eminence of your right hand, press on the back of the fingers of your left hand (fig. 20.11). Pressure is applied through the index finger, supported by the middle and ring fingers, of the left hand (fig 20.12). The alternate sawing motion is initiated by the right hand, allowing the fingers of the left hand to maintain full proprioceptive sensitivity. Work from the lateral margin of the true ribs to just short of the xiphoid process: the first pass is immediately inferior to the costal margin; the second, about 1 inch below that. Be careful not to press on the xiphoid process or the floating ribs. It is important to maintain firm support on the rib cage with your right hand to prevent protective splinting. (2 times).

6. Spleen/Rib Mobilization

Deepening your Front Stance, firmly support the antero-lateral aspect of the right side of the rib cage with the full palmar contact of your widespread left hand. Your right hand makes full and widespread contact with the antero-lateral aspect of the left side of the rib cage (fig. 20.13). A rhythmic pumping movement is initiated by the right hand, while the left hand restricts the free movement of the thorax. On the right (liver) side, the pumping action is up and down, while on the left (spleen) side, the pumping movement is from side to side. Continue pumping until freedom of movement is achieved.

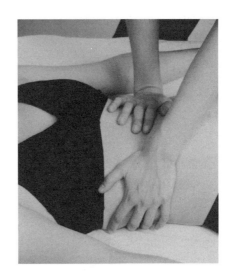

Fig. 20.13

7. Stomach Sawing

Moving into a cephalic Front Stance, use the lateral portion of the palm of the right hand to support the antero-lateral aspect of the left side of the rib cage. With the radial margin of the first three fingers of your left hand, use a sawing motion to sedate the left infracostal region from the xiphoid process to the tenth rib (fig. 20.14). Then apply pressure with the thenar eminence of your right hand through the fingers of the left hand (fig. 20.15). Perform this movement two times: the first pass is immediately inferior to the costal margin; the second, about 1 inch below that. It is important to maintain firm support on the rib cage with the fingers of your right hand to prevent protective splinting. Be careful not to press on the floating ribs or the xiphoid process. (Be mindful of people who have eaten recently—the pressure employed must be much lighter or omitted entirely.) (2 times.)

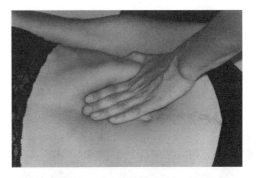

Fig. 20.14

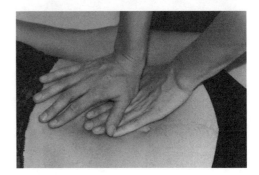

Fig. 20.15

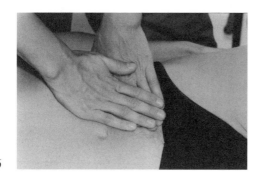

Fig. 20.16

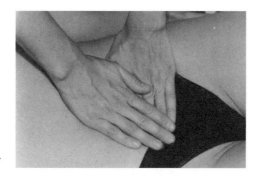

Fig. 20.17

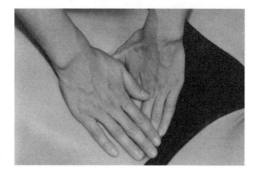

Fig. 20.18

8. Pelvic Basin

Move toward the pelvis, maintaining a caudal Front Stance. Beginning at the left ASIS, apply circular compressions with the pads of the fingers of your left hand, tracing a triangular area from the left ASIS to just above the pubic bone and over to the right ASIS (figs. 20.16, 20.17, 20.18). Then return in a straight line, below the umbilicus, to the left ASIS. Use hand-over-hand pressure to maximize the proprioceptive sensitivity of your treating hand. Increase the pressure in the second pass. (2 times.)

9. Conception Vessel

Assume a Balanced Stance at the pelvis. Bend the fingers of the left hand at the junction of the second and third phalanges so that the tips of all four fingers are even (fig. 20.19), and place on the linea alba at the superior margin of the pubic bone. Apply pressure with your right palm over the knuckles of your left hand, from the pubic bone to just below the xiphoid process (fig. 20.20). Create a rolling motion with your left hand, from inferior to superior, as if you were squeezing a tube of toothpaste. Be careful not to compress directly over the umbilicus or the xiphoid process. The heel of the left hand and the fingers of the right hand provide a steady, balancing pressure on both rectus muscles simultaneously to prevent protective splinting. Use pressure to client's tolerance level. (2 times.)

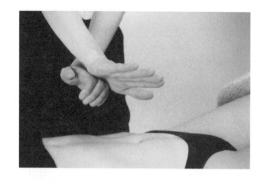

Fig. 20.19

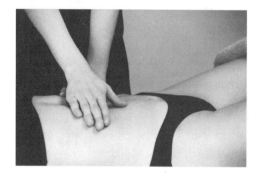

Fig. 20.20

10. Stomach Meridian (bilateral)

Maintaining the same body and hand positions, place your hands on the Stomach Meridian on the right side, 2 inches lateral to the linea alba in the middle of the abdominal rectus muscle (figs. 20.21, 20.22). Apply the same rolling motion described in step 9 from the inferior costal margin to the pubic ramus. Press to client's tolerance level. Repeat on the Stomach Meridian pathway on the left. Lighten your pressure at the ovaries. (2 times.)

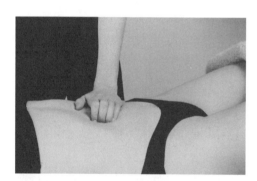

Fig. 20.21

11. Abdominal Rocking

Finish with Abdominal Rocking as described in step 2 on page 178. Because the abdomen is so rarely manipulated, invite your client to notice the change in abdominal tension resulting from your treatment.

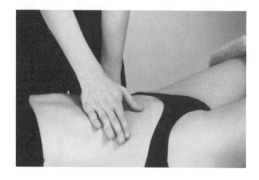

Fig. 20.22

Practice Outline

The Abdomen

1. Lumbar Oscillation	Cephalic Front Stance	Until unrestricted
2. Abdominal Rocking	Balanced Stance	10-15 times
3. Large Intestine	Balanced Stance	3 times
4. Liver/Rib Mobilization	Cephalic Front Stance	Until unrestricted
5. Liver Sawing	Cephalic Front Stance	2 times
6. Spleen/Rib Mobilization	Deep Front Stance	Until unrestricted
7. Stomach Sawing	Cephalic Front Stance	2 times
8. Pelvic Basin	Caudal Front Stance	2 times
9. Conception Vessel	Balanced Stance	2 times
10. Stomach Meridian (bilateral)	Balanced Stance	2 times
11. Abdominal Rocking	Until unrestricted	

CHAPTER 21

TREATMENT OF THE CHEST AND ARMS

1. Bilateral Rib Mobilization

Stand at your client's left side, near the waist, in a cephalic Front Stance (fig. 21.1). Place your left hand on the lower right ribs and your right hand on the lower left ribs (costal 7, 8, and 9) (fig. 21.2). Alternately pump with one hand and restrict with the other, gradually working up the rib cage to the infraclavicular margin and back down to the lower ribs. Do not exert pressure on women's breasts. (1 time up and down.)

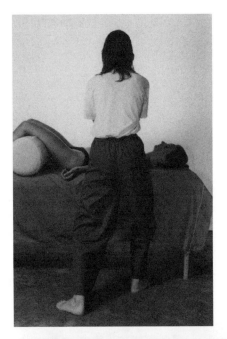

Fig. 21.1

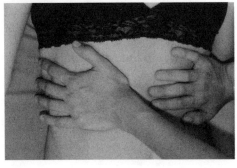

Fig. 21.2

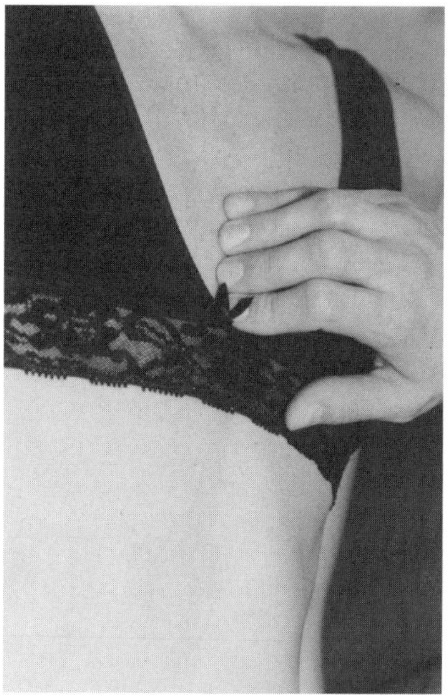

2. Conception Vessel—Sternum

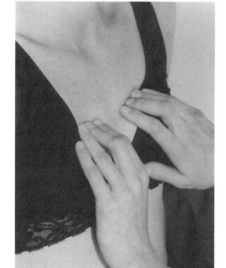

Fig. 21.3

Step up to the lower costal margin in a closed cephalic Front Stance. Place the pads of the first three fingers of your right hand on the inferior sternal centerline (fig. 21.3). The left hand maintains neutral contact with the abdomen. Perform alternate compressive frictions up the sternal midline, moving inferior to superior. Pay special attention to the Heart Envelope Mu Point (CV17) between the fourth and fifth ribs; begin pressure very lightly here as this point can be extremely sensitive. Take care not to compress directly over the xiphoid process, and be careful that your movements don't irritate your client's chest hairs. (2 times.)

3. Sternal Margin (bilateral)

Maintaining the same stance, place your fingers on the sternal margins. With the pads of your first three fingers, apply bilateral compressive circular frictions up the costosternal margins, from the base of the sternum to the clavicles (fig. 21.4). Pressure is focused between the ribs. (2 times.)

Fig. 21.4

4. Pectorals (bilateral)

Maintaining your cephalic Front Stance, place the pads of your first three fingers on the pectoralis major at the sternoclavicular margin (fig. 21.5). Apply bilateral circular frictions, medial to lateral, from the sternal insertion of the pectoralis to the fifth anterior vertical line at the deltoid margin, moving progressively downward with each pass until you have covered the top two-thirds of the pectoralis muscle. The number of passes depends on the size of your client's chest. Begin lightly and work deeper, being cautious of extra sensitivity at the Lung Mu points, 1 inch below the infraclavicular fossa. Do not apply pressure to breast tissue. (2 times.)

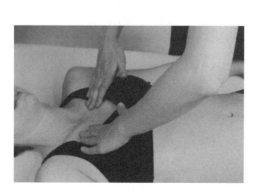

Fig. 21.5

5. Deltoid Margin (bilateral)

Maintaining the same stance, place broad thumbs in the supero-medial margin of the deltopectoral groove (fig. 21.6). Apply bilateral compressions along the deltoid margin to the biceps. (2 times.)

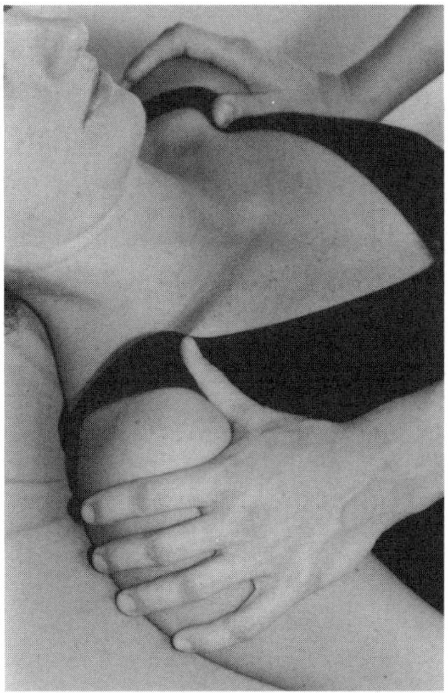

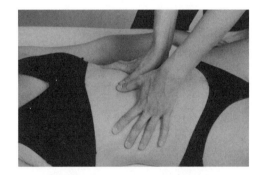

Fig. 21.6

6. Intercostals (bilateral)

Maintaining your cephalic Front Stance, move toward your client's waist. Place your little fingers in the tenth intercostal space, with your other fingers fanned over the adjoining intercostal spaces (fig. 21.7). Use broad fingers to apply compressive frictions, medial to lateral, to release the intercostal muscles. Repeat, moving your hands superior to begin with your little finger at the seventh intercostal space. If your client is very ticklish, this technique may not be possible. Do not apply compression to breast tissue. (2 times.)

Fig. 21.7

7. Infracostal Margin (bilateral)

Maintain your stance. Spreading your hands widely for proprioceptive cueing, use very broad thumbs to bilaterally compress the inferior border of the rib cage (fig. 21.8). Begin on either side of the xiphoid process, continuing to the lateral margin of the false ribs. Do not compress the floating ribs. Initially contact is at the inferior edge of the costochondral border, but the compressions then roll under the rib cage to release the anterior insertions of the diaphragm. Be mindful of prior rib injuries. If your client defends with protective splinting (see page 122), stop the compressions. (2 times.)

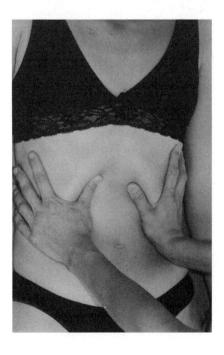

Fig. 21.8

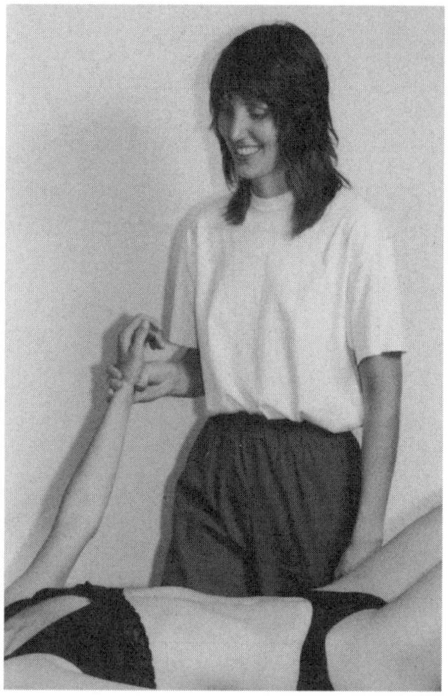

8. Pectoralis Tendon and Medial Deltoid

Move toward the mid-chest in a cephalic Front Stance. Move your client's left arm to a 90-degree angle sideways. Grasp your client's left wrist with your right hand and oscillate the arm until it releases (fig. 21.9). Using the heel of your left hand, knead the pectoral insertion and then use your full hand to knead the anterior and medial heads of the deltoid, proximal to distal (fig. 21.10). (2 times.)

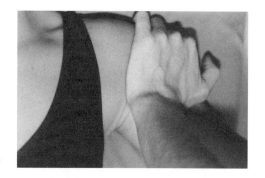

Fig. 21.9

Fig. 21.10

9. Biceps Sawing

Move deeper into the same stance and continue to hold the wrist. Place the back of your client's arm on the table at a 45-degree angle to his or her body, with the forearm flexed at 90 degrees (fig. 21.11). The client's wrist is held by your right hand. With the palm of your left hand, apply a sawing movement down the medial side and up the lateral side of the biceps (fig. 21.12). The part of the biceps being accessed is controlled by your movement of the client's forearm at the wrist. The medial aspect of the biceps is compressed by the heel of your treating hand, the lateral aspect by the heads of your metacarpals. (2 times.)

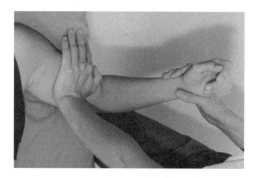

Fig. 21.11

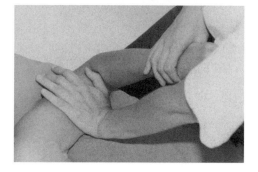

Fig. 21.12

10. Heart Meridian—Anterior Forearm

Close your Front Stance and move down to the hip. Straighten your client's arm and rest it on the table. Support the arm at the wrist with your left hand and apply compressions with your right thumb from the elbow crease, along the Heart Meridian, to the wrist crease (fig. 21.13). Use firm, broad, ball-of-thumb pressure. (2 times.)

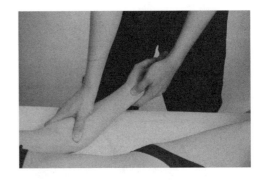

Fig. 21.13

11. Heart Envelope Meridian—Anterior Forearm

Maintaining the same stance, switch support of the wrist to your right hand (fig. 21.14). If the arm does not extend easily, lift the arm slightly to ease pressure at the elbow. Apply compressions with your left hand from the elbow crease, along the Heart Envelope Meridian, to the wrist crease. Use firm, broad, ball-of-thumb pressure. (2 times.)

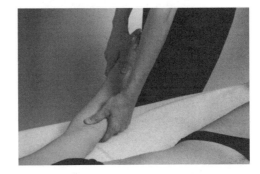

Fig. 21.14

12. Lung Meridian—Anterior Forearm

Continuing to support the wrist with your right hand, move into an open Front Stance and slightly abduct the arm (fig. 21.15). Apply compressions with your left hand along the Lung Meridian, from the elbow crease to the wrist crease. Use firm, broad ball-of-thumb pressure. (2 times.)

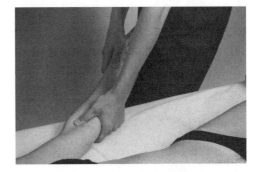

Fig. 21.15

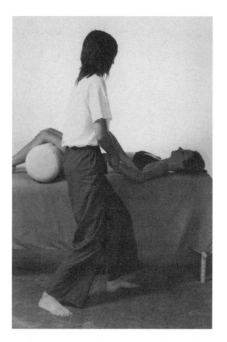

Fig. 21.16

13. Small Intestine Meridian— Posterior Forearm

Maintaining the same stance, pronate your client's forearm by moving the elbow laterally, with a flipping motion, to accommodate restricted movement in the glenohumeral joint (fig. 21.16). Continue to support your client's wrist with your right hand. Apply compressions with your left hand along the Small Intestine Meridian, from the carpo-ulnar fossa (distal to the wrist crease) to the lateral epicondyle of the humerus at the elbow crease (fig. 21.17). Use firm, broad ball-of-thumb pressure. (2 times.)

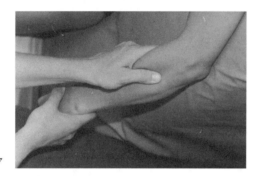

Fig. 21.17

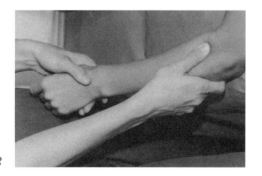

Fig. 21.18

14. Triple Heater Meridian— Posterior Forearm

Maintaining your stance, switch support of the prone wrist to your left hand. Apply compressions with your right hand along the Triple Heater Meridian, from the interstyloid fossa at the wrist crease to the medial aspect of the olecranon process, in line with the elbow crease (fig. 21.18). The Triple Heater Meridian passes lateral to the extensor muscle mass. Use firm ball-of-thumb pressure. (2 times.)

15. Large Intestine Meridian—Posterior Forearm

Assuming a closed Front Stance, continue to support your client's prone wrist with your left hand. Apply compressions with your right hand along the Large Intestine Meridian; begin distal to the styloid process of the radius and continue to the elbow crease (fig. 21.19). Use firm ball-of-thumb pressure. (2 times.)

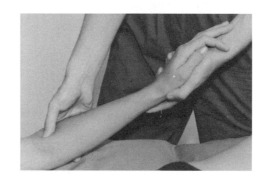

Fig. 21.19

Continue onto the treatment of the hands on the client's left side before switching to the right.

Practice Outline

Chest and Arms

1. Bilateral Rib Mobilization	Cephalic Front Stance	1 time up and down
2. Conception Vessel—Sternum	Closed Cephalic Front Stance	2 times
3. Sternal Margin (bilateral)	Closed Cephalic Front Stance	2 times
4. Pectorals (bilateral)	Closed Cephalic Front Stance	2 times
5. Deltoid Margin (bilateral)	Closed Cephalic Front Stance	2 times
6. Intercostals (bilateral)	Cephalic Front Stance	2 times
7. Infracostal Margin (bilateral)	Cephalic Front Stance	2 times
8. Pectoralis Tendon and Medial Deltoid	Cephalic Front Stance	2 times
9. Biceps Sawing	Deeper Cephalic Front Stance	2 times
10. Heart Meridian—Anterior Forearm	Closed Front Stance	2 times
11. Heart Envelope Meridian—Anterior Forearm	Closed Front Stance	2 times
12. Lung Meridian—Anterior Forearm	Open Front Stance	2 times
13. Small Intestine Meridian—Posterior Forearm	Open Front Stance	2 times
14. Triple Heater Meridian—Posterior Forearm	Open Front Stance	2 times
15. Large Intestine Meridian—Posterior Forearm	Closed Front Stance	2 times

Treat the client's hand (protocol in chapter 22) before switching to treat the hand and arm on the opposite side.

CHAPTER 22

TREATMENT OF THE HANDS

$\mathbf{M}$AINTAIN THE BALANCED STANCE through the full course of treatment on the hand.

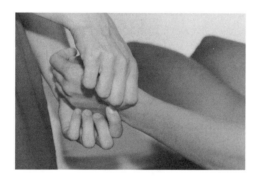

Fig. 22.1

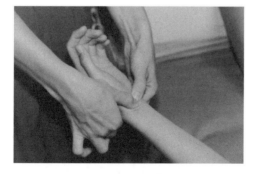

Fig. 22.2

1. Wrist Flip

Standing at the left side in a Balanced Stance, supinate your client's forearm. With the tips of your joined middle fingers supporting your client's arm in the interstyloid fossa (TH4) (fig. 22.1), place your thumbs, tips touching, on the middle of the wrist crease (HE7) (fig. 22.2). Apply traction to the arm and oscillate it to release all of the joints. Create a rapid flipping motion of the wrist by alternately pressing with your thumbs and middle fingers. Perform this action until your client's wrist movement becomes free and unrestricted.

2. Wrist Flop

Wedge the sides of the supine radius and ulna between the pads of your fingers and your thenar eminences (figs. 22.3 [top view], 22.4 [bottom view]). Shake the wrist using rapid, alternating proximo-distal motions, until it flops loosely from side to side. When the fingers loosely strike the inside of your forearms, you will hear a rhythmic popping sound.

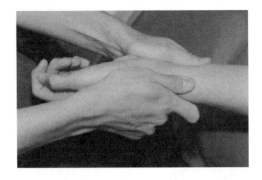

Fig. 22.3

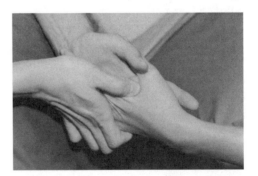

Fig. 22.4

3. Large and Small Intestine Meridian Source Points

Grasp your client's left hand with your left hand as if you were shaking hands. Using your right hand, press your thumbtip and the tip of your middle finger perpendicularly into the medial edge of the second metacarpal and the lateral edge of the fifth metacarpal—feel for the notches on the anterior surfaces of the metacarpals (fig. 22.5). Apply alternate pressure between your thumb and middle finger. (10 times.)

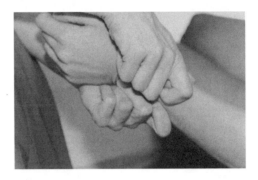

Fig. 22.5

4. Heart Envelope, Heart, and Triple Heater Points

With your thumbs and fingertips, grasp the spaces between the second and third metacarpals and the fourth and fifth metacarpals on either side of your client's left hand (fig. 22.6). Apply compressive frictions first with your left hand, then with your right. (10 times.)

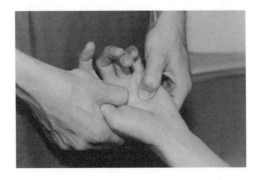

Fig. 22.6

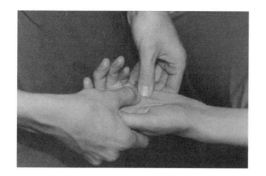

Fig. 22.7

5. Metacarpal Mobilization

Grasp the supine hand between your flat fingertips and the heels of your palms. Place your left thumb on the head of the fifth metacarpal and your right thumb on the head of the fourth metacarpal, both supported on the dorsal surface by the fingertips, and generate a back-and-forth sawing movement (fig. 22.7). Shift your thumb placement to the fourth and third metacarpals, then the third and second, and finally to the second and first. Continue at each interval until the movement of the metacarpals is free and easy.

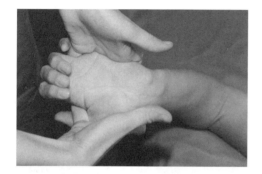

Fig. 22.8

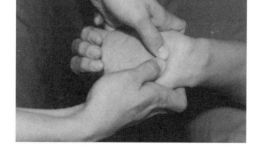

Fig. 22.9

6. Palmar Zones

Grasp the supine hand with the little finger of your right hand hooked between the web of the thumb and index finger, and the little finger of your left hand hooked in the web between the fourth and fifth fingers. Hold the edges of your client's palm between the heads of your metacarpals (fig. 22.8). Take care not to put undue pressure on your client's thumb and little finger metacarpophalangeal joints. Place the tips of your second, third, and fourth fingers on the dorsal surface of your client's hand while spreading the palm with your hooked little fingers. Bring the wrist into full extension.

Starting in the center of the palm, at the heel, apply horizontal compressions with your thumbtips, arching out and down toward the edges of the palm (fig. 22.9). Repeat across 4 or 5 zones from the heel of the hands to the heads of the metacarpals.

Position your hands now at the base of the palm, thumbtips touching. Apply vertical compressions on the palmar midline, from the heel of the hand to the metacarpal heads (figs. 22.10, 22.11). Slide your thumbs apart and repeat compressions between the second and third metacarpals and the fourth and fifth metacarpals, from the heel to the metacarpal heads. Then slide thumbs wider, to the medial and lateral margins of the first and fifth metacarpals, and repeat the vertical compressions. (1 time at each zone.)

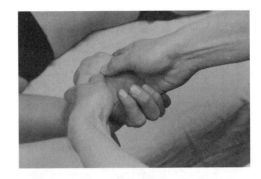

Fig. 22.10

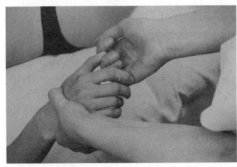

Fig. 22.11

7. Finger Snaps

Pronate your client's hand and grasp the palm with your left hand. Hold the base of the thumb between the middle phalanges of the index and middle fingers of your right hand, with your thumb pressed firmly against your index finger. Apply a spiraling compressive motion from the base of the thumb to the tip (figs. 22.12, 22.13, 22.14). Release with a sharp upward snap (your fingers create an audible pop). Repeat on the other four fingers. (1 time each finger.)

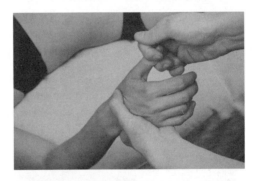

Fig. 22.12

Reverse instructions for treatment of the arms, (chapter 21, steps 8–15), and for treatment of the hands, and repeat on the opposite side.

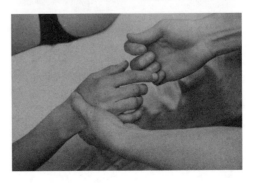

Fig. 22.13

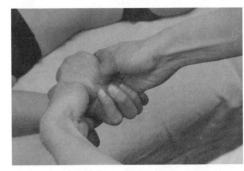

Fig. 22.14

Practice Outline

The Hands

1. Wrist Flip	Balanced Stance	Until unrestricted
2. Wrist Flop	Balanced Stance	
3. Large and Small Intestine Meridian Source Points	Balanced Stance	10 times
4. Heart Envelope, Heart, and Triple Heater Points	Balanced Stance	10 times
5. Metacarpal Mobilization	Balanced Stance	Until unrestricted
6. Palmar Zones (horizontal and vertical)	Balanced Stance	1 time each zone
7. Finger Snaps	Balanced Stance	1 time each finger

Reverse instructions for treatment of the arm (chapter 21, steps 8–15) and treatment of the hand, and perform on the opposite side.

CHAPTER 23

TREATMENT OF THE ANTERIOR LEGS

BECAUSE YOU HAVE treated first the left arm and then the right arm, you now begin treatment with the right leg since you are already on that side.

1. Gallbladder Meridian—Thigh

Face the middle of your client's right thigh in a Balanced Stance (fig. 23.1). Apply pressure with both hands, thumbtips touching, from the inferior margin of the greater trochanter, along the course of the tensor fasciae latae, to the lateral epicondyle of the femur (fig. 23.2). First apply perpendicular pressure into the tensor fasciae latae, then press at a 45-degree angle upward into the vastus lateralis. Shift your weight from your cephalic to your caudal leg to keep your center of gravity aligned with your thumbs. Use a broad thumb with gentle pressure. (2 times.)

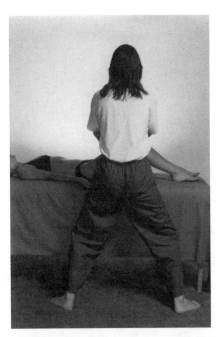

Fig. 23.1

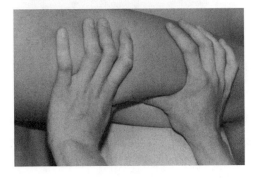

Fig. 23.2

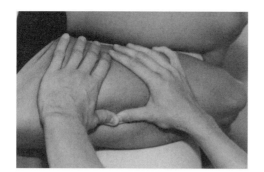

Fig. 23.3

2. Stomach Meridian—Thigh

Move to your client's knee and shift into a cephalic Front Stance. With your left hand supporting the leg at the hip in neutral rotation, apply pressure with your right hand, beginning 1½ inches below the ASIS, at the convergence of the tensor fasciae latae and the sartorius (fig. 23.3). Continue with both hands along the antero-lateral margin of the quadriceps to the superior lateral margin of the patella. Shifting between a cephalic Front Stance and a cephalic Back Stance in order to keep your center of gravity aligned with your thumbs, compress perpendicular to the quadriceps cylinder, using firm ball-of-thumb pressure. (2 times.)

3. Spleen Meridian—Thigh

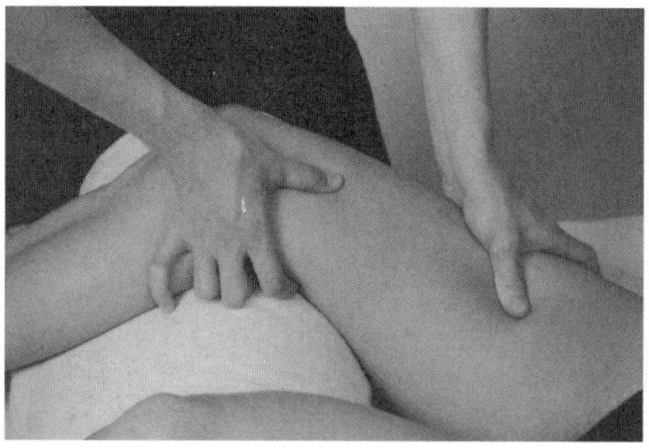

Continue standing at the knee in a cephalic Back Stance. With your right hand supporting the leg at the knee in slight lateral rotation, apply pressure with your left hand from the inferior head of the vastus medialis, along the antero-medial margin of the quadriceps, to just below the inguinal ligament at the femoral artery (fig. 23.4). Shifting between a cephalic Back Stance and a cephalic Front Stance in order to keep your center of gravity aligned with your thumbs, compress perpendicular to the vastus medialis cylinder. Use a broad thumb. As this is a Yin meridian, be especially gentle. (2 times.)

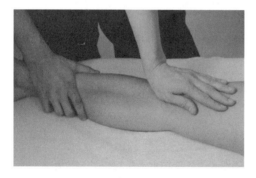

Fig. 23.4

4. Patella Circumduction

Rotate to a closed cephalic Front Stance. With your right hand supporting the leg at the distal end of the tibia, apply palmar circumduction with your left hand to the patella in both directions (fig. 23.5). Make sure that the patella moves freely. (3 times.)

In the same position, support either side of the knee with the fingers of both hands under the popliteal fossa (fig. 23.6). Apply simultaneous bilateral compressions in a semicircle, from the superior to the inferior edge of the patella, using the balls of your thumbs. (2 times.)

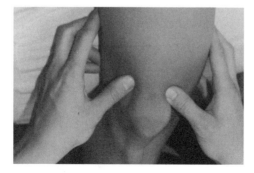

Fig. 23.5

Fig. 23.6

5. Gallbladder Meridian—Lower Leg

Stand midway between the knee and the foot in a Balanced Stance. Support your client's leg in medial rotation with your left hand at the knee. Apply pressure with your right hand along the course of the peroneus longus from the head of the fibula to the hollow antero-inferior to the lateral malleolus (fig. 23.7). Shift your weight from your cephalic to your caudal leg to keep your center of gravity aligned with your thumbs. Compress perpendicular to the peroneal cylinder, using firm ball-of-thumb pressure. (2 times.)

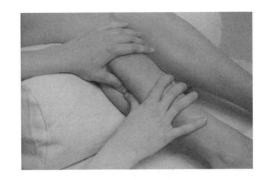

Fig. 23.7

6. Stomach Meridian—Lower Leg

Move to your client's ankle and shift into a cephalic Front Stance. With your left hand supporting the leg at the knee in neutral rotation, apply pressure with your right hand from just below the lateral epicondyle of the tibia, ¼ inch lateral to the bone on the tibialis anterior, to the tibio-taler fossa (fig. 23.8). Shifting between a cephalic Front Stance and a cephalic Back Stance in order to keep your center of gravity aligned with your thumbs, compress perpendicular to the cylinder of the tibialis anterior, using firm ball-of-thumb pressure. (2 times.)

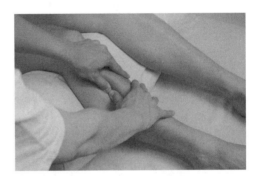

Fig. 23.8

7. Spleen and Liver Meridians— Lower Leg

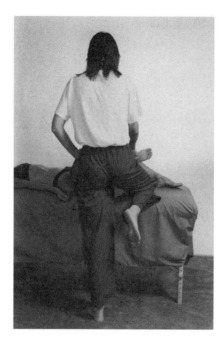

Fig. 23.9

Standing at the knee, flex your client's leg at the knee and hip, and abduct it. Either using a bolster or with your right knee on the table for support, rest your client's knee against your right thigh or on the bolster, drawing the foot in toward the groin (fig. 23.9). With your left hand resting on the leg at the knee, apply pressure with your right hand simultaneously along the center of the tibial plateau and the medial edge of the tibia (fig. 23.10). Compress perpendicular to the middle of the tibial plateau with the head of your second metacarpal; simultaneously press perpendicular and in, hooking under the medial edge of the tibia with your thumb in a can-opener-like movement. The compression moves from the medial malleolus to the medial epicondyle of the tibia. As these are Yin meridians, pressure is especially gentle. (2 times.) **Caution:** This movement is contraindicated for pregnant women.

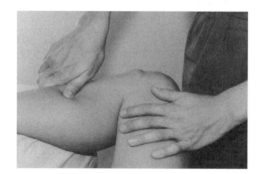

Fig. 23.10

8. Liver Meridian—Thigh

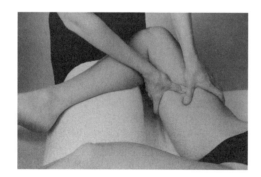

Fig. 23.11

Supporting the leg in the same position, shift your left leg and your body weight cephalad. With your thumbs interwoven, apply pressure from the medial epicondyle of the femur along the medial aspect of the thigh to just below the inguinal crease (fig. 23.11). Simultaneously compress all surfaces of the adductor muscle group. Use very broad and gentle thumbs. (2 times.)

9. Adductor Stretch and Saw

Maintaining support of the leg, shift your body weight caudal. Rest the palm of your right hand on the ASIS of the opposite hip for stabilization, then gently press the knee toward the table. This is an extended range-of-motion stretch—be very mindful of overly tight adductors. After stretching, continue supporting the knee with your leg if necessary; then, stabilizing the knee with your left hand, apply sawing compressions with your right palm from the medial epicondyle of the femur, along the midline of the medial aspect of the thigh, to just below the inguinal crease (fig. 23.12). Go upward in one pass and downward in the second. (2 times.)

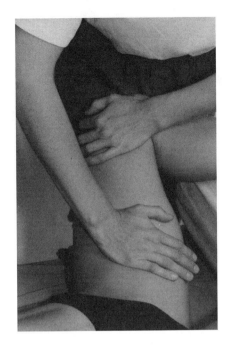

Fig. 23.12

Reverse instructions and treat the opposite leg.

Practice Outline

Anterior Legs

1. Gallbladder Meridian—Thigh	Balanced Stance	2 times
2. Stomach Meridian—Thigh	Cephalic Front to Back Stance	2 times
3. Spleen Meridian—Thigh	Cephalic Back to Front Stance	2 times
4. Patella Circumduction	Closed Cephalic Front Stance	Circumduction—3 times
		Semicircular compressions —2 times
5. Gallbladder Meridian— Lower Leg	Balanced Stance	2 times
6. Stomach Meridian— Lower Leg	Cephalic Front to Back Stance	2 times
7. Spleen and Liver Meridians— Lower Leg	Supporting client's leg	2 times
8. Liver Meridian—Thigh	Supporting client's leg	2 times
9. Adductor Stretch and Saw	Supporting client's leg	2 times (once up and once down)

Reverse instructions to treat the opposite leg.

CHAPTER 24

SEATED SHIATSU

THE TECHNIQUES DESCRIBED in this chapter should be applied in the following order: (1) work each point in sequence (Gb21, TH15, SI14, and SI15) on one shoulder, then repeat the sequence twice more on the same side; (2) work each periscapular pathway three times in sequence; and finally (3) perform the same sequences on the opposite side.

Work both shoulders before treating the neck. When working the neck, treat the points Bl10 and Gb20 in sequence three times before treating the cervical pathways. Perform range-of-motion stretching, and end your treatment with *kyo ku te* (hand music).

To obtain the maximum benefit without unduly tiring yourself, be sure that your client's chair is low enough for you to make efficient use of gravity.

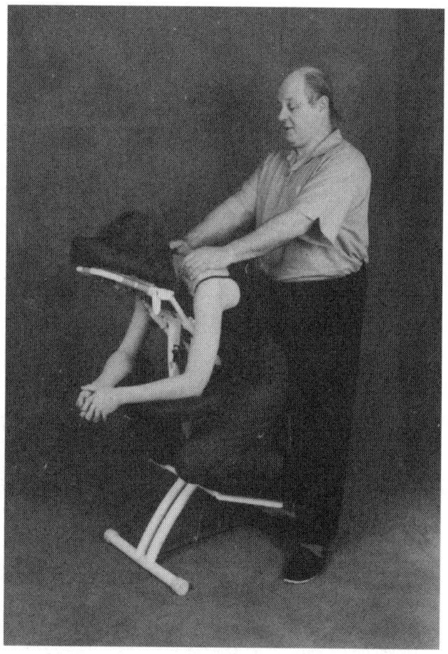

Fig. 24.1

SHOULDERS

1. Shoulder Shaking

Standing in a Front Stance behind your seated client, firmly grasp both shoulders (fig. 24.1). Be careful to use the flat part of your hand, as the anterior deltoid region can be very sensitive to poking pressure. Alternately oscillate the shoulders until they drop and move freely.

2. Suprascapular Points

A. Gallbladder 21, the motor release point for the medial head of the trapezius, lies on the medio-lateral and antero-posterior midline of the medial head of the trapezius (fig. 24.2). Standing in a Front Stance in front of your seated client (fig. 24.3), place your index finger on the junction of the trapezius and the anterior neck muscles; then place your fourth finger on the acromion process. Your middle finger falls between them in the middle of the lateral midline of the medial head of the trapezius. With your fingers spread wide for proprioceptive cueing, make sure that your treating thumb is in the antero-posterior midline (fig. 24.4). Be careful—the superior tubercle of the coracoid process of the scapula, which lies just lateral and posterior to Gb21, is very sensitive to pressure. If the point feels hard as bone, it probably is bone, in which case you should continue searching for the acupoint. Apply thumb-over-thumb pressure (fig. 24.5) for 10 seconds, or for as long as it takes to effect an adequate release.

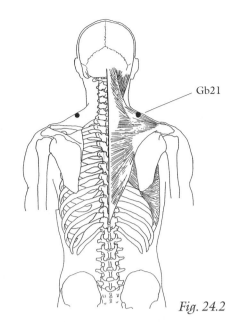

Fig. 24.2

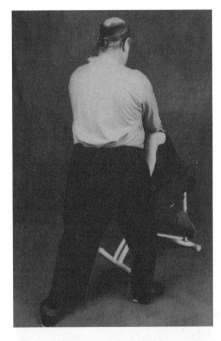

Fig. 24.3

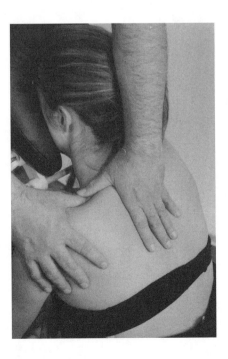

Fig. 24.5

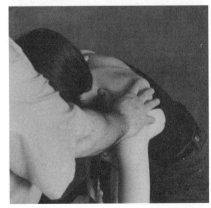

Fig. 24.4

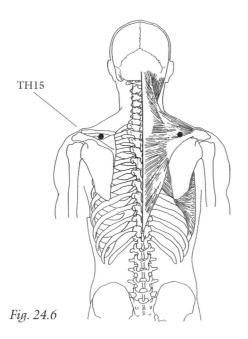

TH15

Fig. 24.6

B. Triple Heater 15 is the motor release point for the supraspinatus (fig. 24.6). It is located 1 acu-inch below Gb21, in the middle of the supraspinatus. Standing behind your client, slide your thumb directly inferior 1 acu-inch from Gb21 (fig. 24.7). You will feel a groove, or striation, in the tissue. Apply thumb-over-thumb pressure at a 45-degree angle down into the supraspinatus fossa for 10 seconds (fig. 24.8).

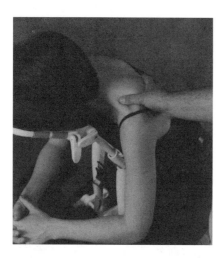

Fig. 24.7

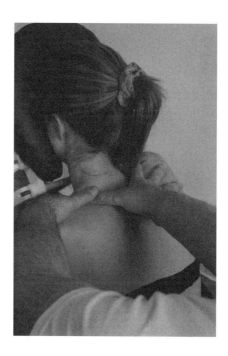

Fig. 24.8

C. Small Intestine 14 is the origin release point for the levator scapulae (fig. 24.9). This point is located just supero-medial to the medial superior angle of the scapula, in a space between the second and third ribs. Find the levator scapula tendon, then delicately probe for the acupoint (fig. 24.10). Apply thumb-over-thumb pressure perpendicularly into the point for 10 seconds (fig. 24.11).

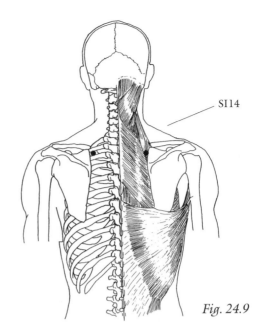

SI14

Fig. 24.9

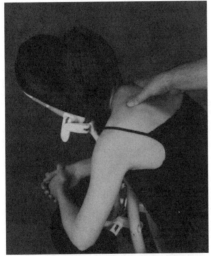

Fig. 24.10

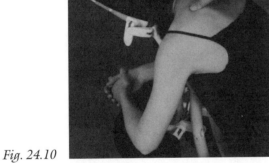

Fig. 24.11

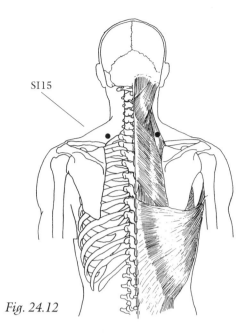

SI15

Fig. 24.12

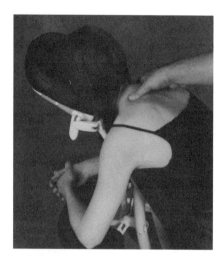

Fig. 24.13

D. Small Intestine 15, the motor release point for the levator scapulae, forms an equilateral triangle with TH15 and SI14 (fig. 24.12). With your middle fingertip on TH15 and your thumb on SI14, gently feel for a dimple with your forefinger at the apex of this would-be triangle and then apply pressure with your thumb (fig. 24.13). Pressure is thumb-over-thumb, perpendicular to the point, for 10 seconds (fig. 24.14).

Press these points—Gb21, TH15, SI14, and SI15—in sequence. Then repeat the entire sequence 2 more times. Go on to treat the meridian pathways (steps 3–5) that run through the shoulder area, then repeat steps 2-5 on the opposite side.

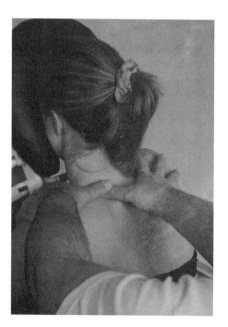

Fig. 24.14

3. Seki Sai Sen (Thoracic)

Maintaining your Front Stance, with your thumb-tip between the spinous process of T5 and T6, apply perpendicular entry-level pressure into the lamina groove between the two spinous processes (fig. 24.15). Then press at a 45-degree angle into the erector spinae cylinder. Work up to T1, using firm thumb-over-thumb pressure (fig. 24.16). (3 times.)

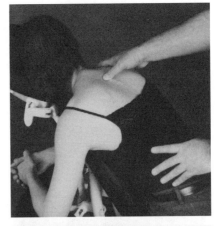

Fig. 24.15

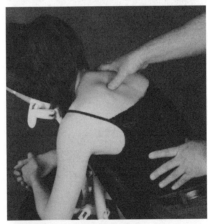

Fig. 24.16

4. Bladder 1 Meridian—Medial Trapezius

Maintaining the same stance, apply pressure to the Bladder 1 meridian on the middle of the erector spinae, from T5 at mid-scapulae level, to T1 (fig. 24.17). Then work out along the top of the medial trapezius to the acromion process. Use firm thumb-over-thumb pressure, perpendicular to the back on Bl1 (fig. 24.18); then switch to a caudal perpendicular vector on the trapezius. Shift your stance laterally around the shoulder so that you can maintain your line of drive. (3 times.)

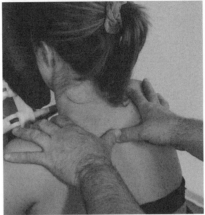

Fig. 24.17

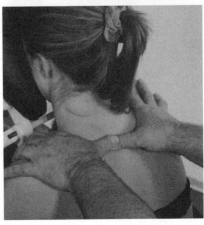

Fig. 24.18

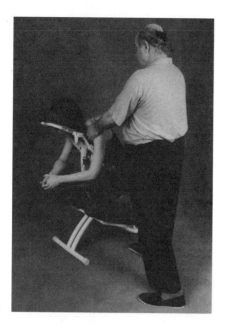

Fig. 24.19

5. Bladder 2 Meridian—Supraspinatus

Shift to a more lateral Front Stance at the side of your client's shoulder (fig. 24.19). Apply pressure along the medial edge of the scapula, from T5 to T3, at a 45-degree angle medially into the erector spinae cylinder (fig. 24.20). Then move laterally along the supraspinous fossa to the end of the scapular spine, pressing 45 degrees caudal (fig. 24.21). Use firm thumb-over-thumb pressure. (3 times.)

Reverse instructions and perform steps 2 through 5 on the client's opposite side.

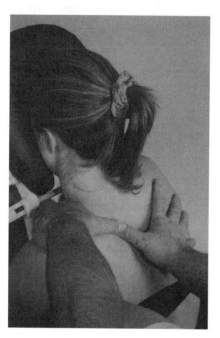

Fig. 24.20

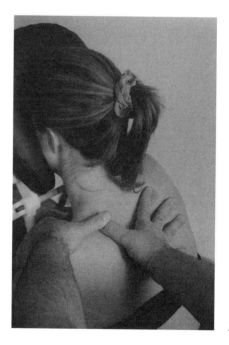

Fig. 24.21

Practice Outline

Seated Shiatsu—Shoulders

1. Shoulder Shaking	Front Stance	Until mobile
2. Suprascapular Points, in sequence:	Front Stance	3 times
A. Gallbladder 21		
B. Triple Heater 15		
C. Small Intestine 14		
D. Small Intestine 15		
3. Seki Sai Sen (Thoracic)	Front Stance	3 times
4. Bladder 1 Meridian—Medial Trapezius	Front Stance	3 times
5. Bladder 2 Meridian—Supraspinatus	Lateral Front Stance	3 times

**Reverse instructions and perform steps
2 through 5 on the opposite side.**

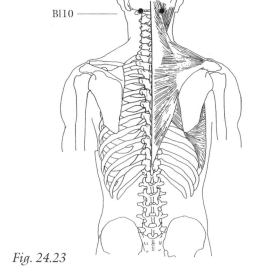

Fig. 24.22

Fig. 24.23

Bl10

6. Suboccipital Points

A. Bladder 10. Standing in a lateral Front Stance behind your client, spread the fingers of your left hand wide on the left rib cage for support. With the ball of your right thumb compress Bladder 10, located on the occiput on the lateral margin of the trapezius insertion (figs. 24.22, 24.23). Use firm and steady pressure for 10 seconds. Compress alternately with Gallbladder 20 (see below). (3 times.)

B. Gallbladder 20. Slide your thumb laterally to GB20, ½ inch below the apex of the notch between the mastoid process and occiput, on line with Bladder 10 (figs. 24.24, 24.25). Compress toward the contralateral eye, using the ball of your thumb. Use firm and steady pressure for 10 seconds. Compress alternately with Bl10. (3 times.)

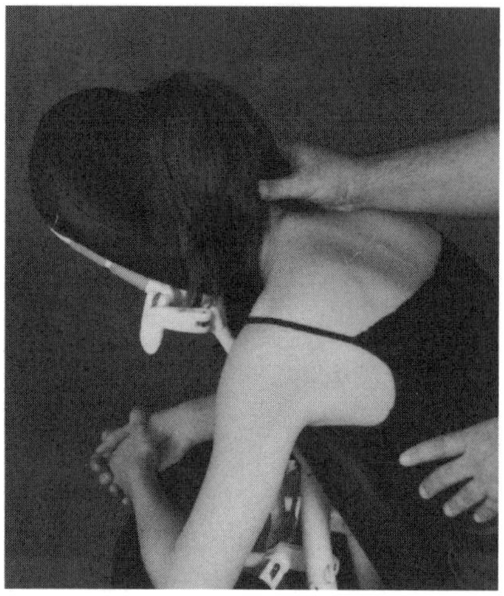

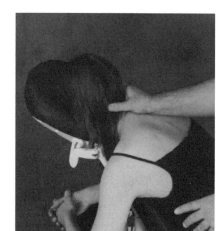

Fig. 24.24

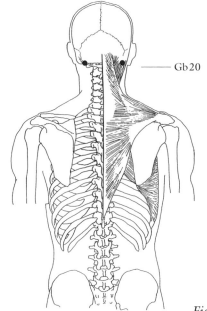

Gb20

Fig. 24.25

7. Cervical Pathways

A. Seki Sai Sen. Stand in a Front Stance facing your client's left shoulder. Place your right thumb on the nuchal line on the client's left side, just lateral to C2; use the thumbtip to apply entry-level pressure into the lamina groove (fig. 24.26, 24.27). Then press 45 degrees lateral into the erector spinae cylinder. Work down the spine between the spinous processes, to the cervico-thoracic junction, using firm pressure for 1 to 3 seconds. (3 times.)

B. Bladder Meridian. Maintaining the same body and hand position, apply compressions with the ball of your right thumb from the occiput down the latero-posterior edge of the superior head of the trapezius (figs. 24.28, 24.29). Move in ½-inch intervals to the base of the neck (C7). Use a firm ball-of-thumb pressure perpendicular to the cylinder of the cervical trapezius. Hold each compression for 1 to 3 seconds. (3 times.)

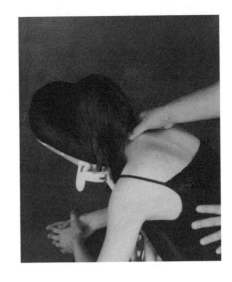

Fig. 24.26

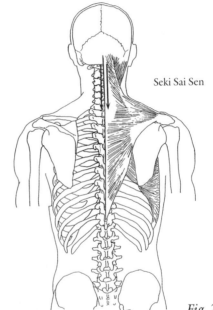

Seki Sai Sen

Fig. 24.27

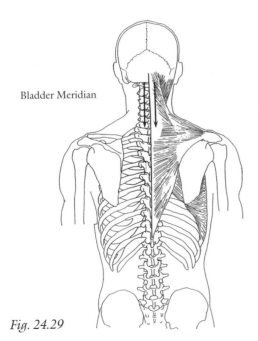

Bladder Meridian

Fig. 24.29

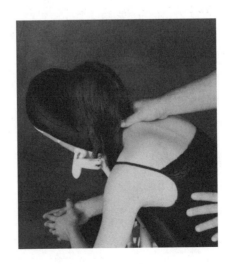

Fig. 24.28

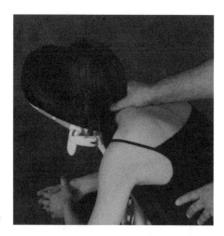

Fig. 24.30

C. Gallbladder Meridian. Maintaining the same body and hand position, apply compressions with the ball of your right thumb from the notch between the mastoid process and the occiput, level with Bl10, to the base of the neck (figs. 24.30, 24.31). Use the posterior aspect of the transverse processes as your deep landmark. Compress at a 45-degree angle toward the opposite eye with firm ball-of-thumb pressure. Hold each compression for 1 to 3 seconds. (3 times.)

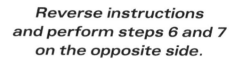

*Reverse instructions
and perform steps 6 and 7
on the opposite side.*

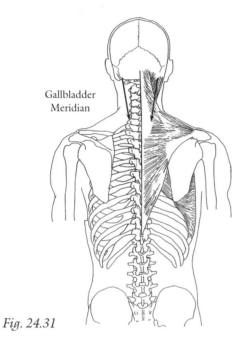

Gallbladder
Meridian

Fig. 24.31

Practice Outline

Seated Shiatsu—Neck

6. Suboccipital Points	Lateral Front Stance	3 times alternately
A. Bladder 10		
B. Gallbladder 20		
7. Cervical Pathways	Front Stance	3 times
A. Seki Sai Sen		
B. Bladder Meridian		
C. Gallbladder Meridian		

*Reverse instructions and perform
steps 6 and 7 on the opposite side.*

EXTENDED RANGE-OF-MOTION STRETCHING

Review the text on range-of-motion stretching on page 163. Have your client sit erect. All left-handed practitioners should reverse left/right instructions.

8. Lateral Stretch

Standing in a lateral Front Stance on the client's left side, cup the parietal prominence with your right hand and anchor the shoulder with your left. Position yourself right up against the back of your client's head, and gently stretch the head and neck up and away from the anchored shoulder (fig. 24.32). The vector of stretch is not directly lateral but more upward and outward. The ideal range of motion for lateral flexion should bring the ear to the shoulder; chronic myofascial shortening will prevent this. Be aware that subluxed, or displaced, vertebrae can cause a painful pinching sensation; if your client indicates pain either verbally or by protective splinting, do not deepen the stretch. Instead, back off slightly and hold for 5 to 10 seconds for neuromuscular accommodation before slowly releasing.

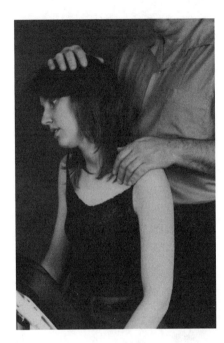

Fig. 24.32

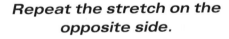

Repeat the stretch on the opposite side.

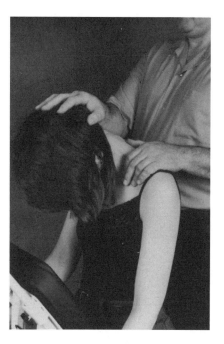

Fig. 24.33

9. Anterior Stretch

Standing in a Front Stance at the center of your client's back, cup the occiput at the nuchal ridge with the heel of your right palm; support the body with your left hand at the shoulder (fig. 24.33). Make sure to cup the shoulder with flat fingers, as the anterior deltoid and pectoralis muscles are quite sensitive to pressure. Stretch the neck by guiding the head upward and outward, flexing the neck so that the chin tips down to the chest. The vector of stretch is upward and out, not forward and down; the intent is to create length between the vertebrae as well as to increase flexion. Do not overstretch and be sure that your client does not feel choked. Continue to hold the stretch for 5 to 10 seconds after you reach the limit of your client's range of motion; this allows for neuromuscular accommodation to the change in tissue resting-length. Instruct the client to be passive during the return to an anatomically neutral posture as you lift their forehead with your right hand.

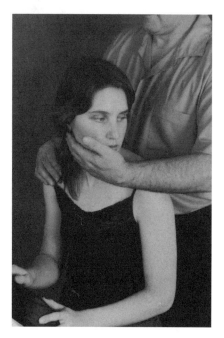

Fig. 24.34

10. Lateral Rotation

Standing slightly behind your client's left side in a Front Stance, support your client's right shoulder with your right hand and cup the right buccal region with your left hand (fig. 24.34). Apply mild traction and slightly extend the neck, rotating the head to the limit of its range of motion; then apply extended range-of-motion stretching. Pressure is evenly distributed between your hands. Do not overstretch. Perform a gentle antero-posterior oscillation if you feel a splinting reflex occur. Hold the extended range-of-motion position for 5 to 10 seconds to allow for neuromuscular accommodation, then slowly release.

Repeat on the opposite side.

11. Manual Traction

Standing behind your client in a Back Stance with your dominant leg behind you, cup the occiput below the nuchal ridge with the heel of your right hand. Place the left hand under the mandible to provide support for the head (fig. 24.35). This hand provides support only—be careful not to constrict the throat in any way. Apply 90 percent of the tractioning pressure with your right hand at the occiput; the left hand only prevents the head and neck from flexing out of your grasp. Sinking low into the Back Stance, wedge your right elbow into your rib cage; then perform the full traction by lifting with your legs. Be careful not to lift with your back; this is a strenuous movement. Apply the traction very slowly. As you reach the limit of spinal extension, you will be counteracting the effects of gravity; the client's weight will begin to hang from the myofascial attachments to the skull, rather than being compressively supported by the intervertebral discs.

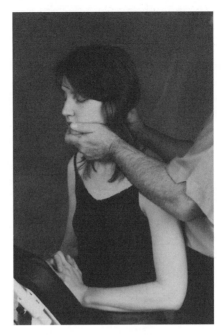

Fig. 24.35

At this point, most people will involuntarily splint to protect their necks. Reassure your client by saying, "Relax your neck and let it stretch. I will support you." As they relax, you will feel the body sink and the spine lengthen. Hold the traction for 5 to 10 seconds, then release very slowly. When the spine regains compressive support, apply lighter traction, this time from your arms, for 5 to 10 seconds longer. Release gently.

Practice Outline

Extended Range-of-Motion Stretching

8. Lateral Stretch	Lateral Front Stance at side	5 to 10 seconds
9. Anterior Stretch	Front Stance	5 to 10 seconds
10. Lateral Rotation	Front Stance	5 to 10 seconds
11. Manual Traction	Back Stance	5 to 10 seconds full traction/ 5 to 10 seconds arm traction

Kyo ku te, or hand music, refers to the rhythmical and musical form of vibration and tapotement movements designed to gently stimulate and balance the sympathetic and parasympathetic nervous systems. The application of these movements will ensure that your client leaves the chair functionally alert and clear. Since meridian-oriented BodyWork Shiatsu promotes the deeply relaxed state of parasympathetic nervous system dominance, hand music is used to prepare your client for reentry to his or her outer environment. If time is not an issue, you can allow your client to rest for five to ten minutes before applying kyo ku te; if there is a time pressure, it can be performed immediately following the range-of-motion stretches.

Kyo ku te is contraindicated in cases of traumatic or chronic injury to the head, neck, or shoulder region. If your client shows an unpleasant reaction of any kind, do not continue. An unpleasant reaction can occur in the presence of high blood pressure; head-, eye-, or toothache; or extreme nervous tension.

All kyo ku te movements require that hands and wrists be flexible; there must be a complete absence of tension or holding in the practitioner's arms and shoulders. Becoming skilled at kyo ku te requires a lot of practice, but the effects are worth the effort. **Note:** Left-handed people should reverse left/right directions.

12. Hammer Fists

Form very loose fists, placing the ball of your thumb over the hole created by your rounded index finger. The fingertips are in very loose contact with the thenar eminence at the base of the thumb, and the thumb lightly touches the middle

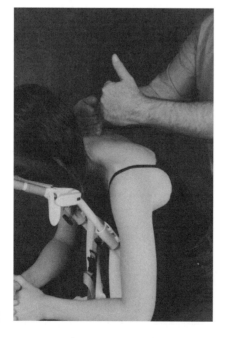

Fig. 24.36

phalangeal joint of the index finger. Your wrists are flexed medially but held very loosely. The movement consists of an alternate drumming up and down the medial and superior aspects of the trapezius (figs. 24.36, 24.37). The motion must be springy and rhythmic, producing a distinct "popping" sound. The lightly bouncing fists produce a gentle stimulation, with no pain.

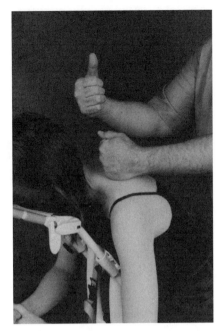

Fig. 24.37

13. Alternate Chopping

With palms facing each other, spread fingers slightly apart. Working on the same area, apply light and springy contact with the ulnar aspect of the little fingers; hands gently brush each other as they alternately rise and fall (figs. 24.38, 24.39). All fingers come together at the moment of contact, then spring apart as contact is released. The combination of the palmar surfaces brushing each other and the fingers bouncing together produces a distinct rustling or crackling sound.

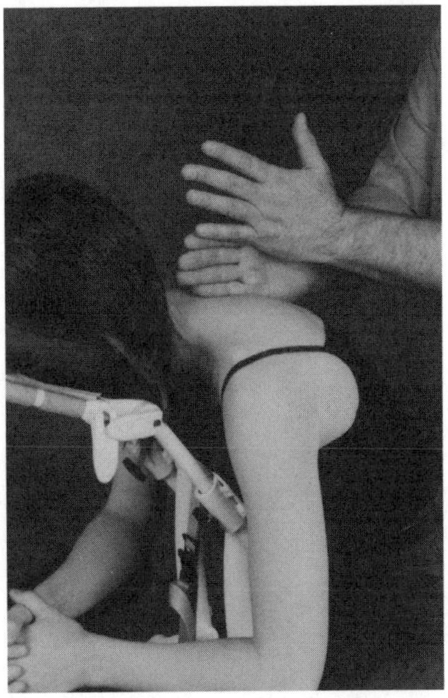

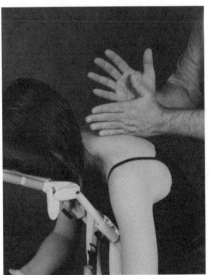

Fig. 24.39

Fig. 24.38

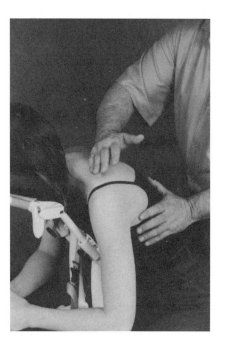

Fig. 24.40

Fig. 24.41

14. Metacarpal Flip-Flops

Contact the same area of the trapezius with the ulnar edge of the fifth metacarpophalangeal joint. All fingers are in light contact with their neighbors; the wrist is slightly flexed. Alternately pronate and supinate your hand in a rapid motion, dragging it along the skin in a cephalic direction from acromion to occiput (figs. 24.40, 24.41). A slapping sound is created by the alternating contacts of the dorsal and palmar surface of your hand on the client's skin. Your treating arm must be adducted, with your elbow leading your hand. The wrist must be entirely free from tension. The shaking is initiated from your shoulder, not your wrist. Perform the motion once up each side.

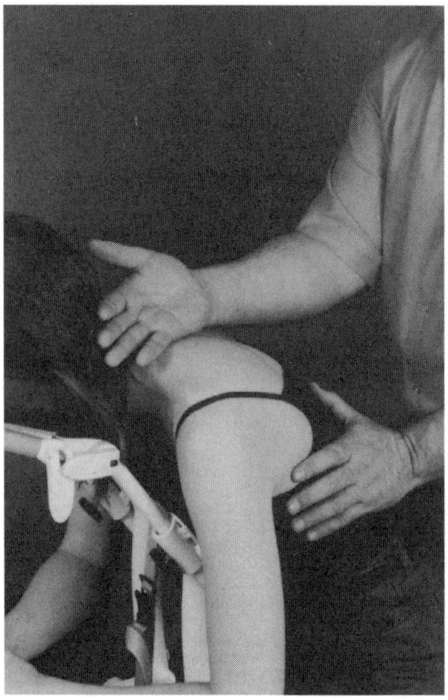

15. Cloud Hands

Form a sphere with your hands as if you were cupping a delicate ball of air. All finger and palm/finger surfaces are in gentle but firm contact. The hands maintain only enough tonus to preserve the sphere. With totally fluid wrists, gently bounce your "cloud" from the acromium, along the posterior aspect of the middle trapezius, to the occiput and back down (figs. 24.42, 24.43). The air rushing out from between the hands at contact produces a soft popping or whooshing sound. Perform once on each side.

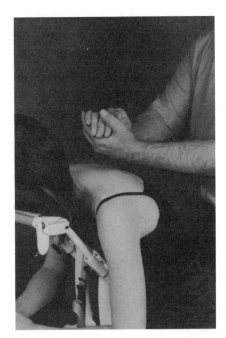

Fig. 24.42

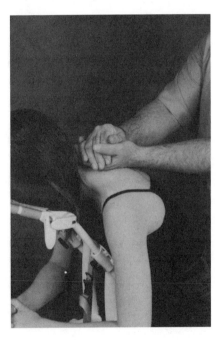

Fig. 24.43

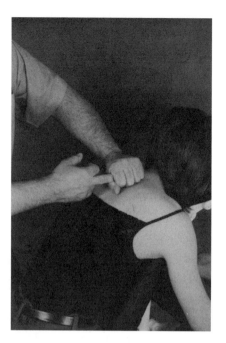

Fig. 24.44

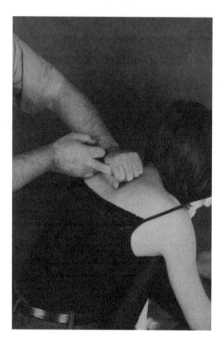

Fig. 24.45

16. Fist and Finger Vibration

Grasp the distal phalanx of the middle finger of your right hand firmly between the index finger and thumb of your left fist. Hold your right hand vertically, midway between pronation and supination. Contact is made directly over the spinous process of the fourth or fifth thoracic vertebra by the dorsal aspect of the middle phalanges of the third, fourth, and fifth fingers of the left hand and the thenar and hypothenar eminences (the lower "eye" of the fist). The index finger and thumb of the left fist tightly clasp the distal phalanx of the middle finger of the vibrating right hand. Make a rapid flexing and extending movement with the right hand from the forearm, while slowly pushing the left hand up the spinous processes to the occiput (figs. 24.44, 24.45, 24.46). A rustling sound is made by the movement of the ulnar aspect of the right hand. (2 times.)

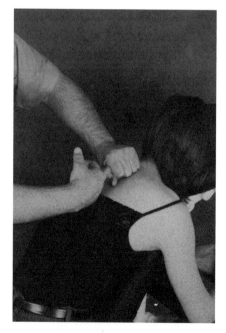

Fig. 24.46

17. Two-Hand Chopping

Place palms firmly together from heel to fingertips, with the fingers spread moderately apart (fig. 24.47). Make a very loose and springy chopping motion, alternately abducting and adducting the wrists (fig. 24.48). Only the edge of the underside of the little finger makes contact with your client. A musical clicking is produced by the fingers slapping together at contact. Treatment is from the acromion to the occiput and back, first one side then the other.

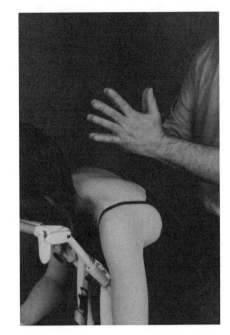

Fig. 24.47

18. Pinch, Shake, and Knead

Grasp the "meat" of the medial heads of the trapezius between the ball of the thumbs and the radial aspect of the middle phalanx of the index finger (fig. 24.49). The grasp should be firm but gentle. Shake the shoulders in alternation to release them, and then gently knead the trapezius. You can signal to your client that the treatment is complete by ending with a pat on the shoulder.

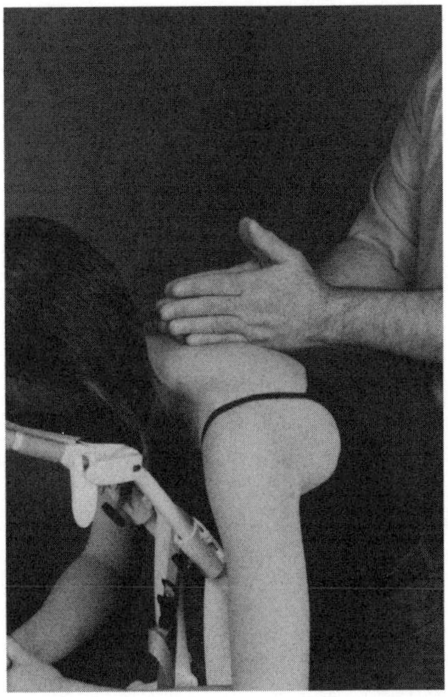

Fig. 24.48

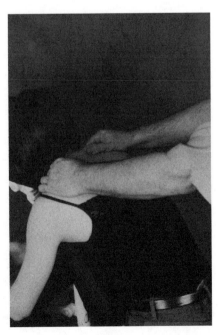

Fig. 24.49

Practice Outline

Kyo Ku Te (Hand Music)

12. Hammer Fists	Loose fists	Drum up and down
13. Alternate Chopping	Fingers slightly apart	Up and down
14. Metacarpal Flip-Flops	Loose wrist	Up and away
15. Cloud Hands	Soft hands	Up and down
16. Fist and Finger Vibration	Vibrating hand, vertical	Vibrate both directions
17. Two-Hand Chopping	Loose wrists	Acromium to occiput
18. Pinch, Shake, and Knead	Gentle grasp	Shake in alternation

APPENDIX 1

CONTRAINDICATIONS AND ENDANGERMENT SITES

"ABOVE ALL, DO NO HARM." This advice, originally given by Hippocrates more than two thousand years ago, still belongs at the beginning of all health-related studies.

Contraindications to therapeutic massage and bodywork in general—and Oriental bodywork therapy in particular—present a very broad and varied reach. Some conditions, such as life-threatening emergencies, should never be approached through the manual therapies. Some conditions, such as pregnancy, require advanced training and experience before Oriental bodywork is safe. And some situations, such as clients under the influence of alcohol, merely require time and a word of caution.

Contraindications also vary according to the hand techniques utilized. Some conditions, such as thrombophlebitis, are totally contraindicated for the fluid-mobilizing techniques such as European massage, and are relatively contraindicated for meridian treatment but require only relative local contraindications for point work. Additionally, certain sites on the body can be endangerment sites under certain circumstances, such as the inside of

the lower legs during the first and third trimesters of pregnancy, and these sites must be differentiated according to technical approach.

In this presentation I have incorporated the considerations of many different approaches to therapeutic massage and bodywork, spanning traditional Western massage, osteopathy, Rolfing, and polarity therapy in addition to Oriental bodywork therapy. I have also incorporated information from such Japanese sources as Serizawa Sensei, Namikoshi Sensei, and Masunaga Sensei.

I will divide contraindications into three categories: absolute contraindications (AC); relative contraindications (RC); and warnings (W). Absolute and relative contraindications will be further differentiated as absolute local contraindications (ALC) and relative local contraindications (RLC). Absolute contraindications refer to conditions that absolutely preclude therapeutic massage and bodywork intervention, regardless of technique or expertise. Relative contraindications refer to conditions that require additional specific training, or other considerations, before they are safe for massage and bodywork. With due consideration, however, these conditions may be treated. Absolute and relative local contraindications will point to site-specific conditions that preclude, or require great care and modification of technique, for the safe use of therapeutic massage and bodywork. Warnings refer to those conditions or situations which only require a word of caution and some consideration, as well as considerations regarding sites of potential endangerment. **Remember: when in doubt—don't!**

ABSOLUTE CONTRAINDICATIONS

Medical Emergencies
Hemorrhage
Shock (all kinds)
Acute, emergency, inflammatory organ disease
  (appendicitis, peritonitis)
Cerebrovascular accident (CVA) (not yet
  stabilized)
Diabetic coma / insulin shock
Epileptic seizure
Myocardial infarction (MI) (not yet stabilized)
Pneumothorax
Severe asthma attack
Lymphangitis (blood poisoning)
Acute poisoning

Very Advanced or Complicated Chronic Organ Diseases
Advanced kidney failure
Advanced respiratory failure
Diabetes with such complications as gangrene,
  advanced heart or kidney disease, or very
  high or unstable blood pressure
Liver failure
Postmyocardial infarction (not yet stabilized)
Postcerebrovascular accident (not yet
  stabilized)

Circulatory Diseases
Severe atherosclerosis
Severe, unstable hypertension

Other Medical Conditions
Eclampsia
Hemophilia
Significant fever (101.5°F/38.35°C)
Systemic / contagious infections
Encephalitis (when symptomatic)

ABSOLUTE LOCAL CONTRAINDICATIONS

Acute Organ Disease
Any inflamed organ
Ectopic pregnancy
Ulcers (peptic, duodenal)

Cancer
Highly metastatic cancers (not yet terminal)

Circulatory
Life-threatening aneurysms (abdominal aorta)
Esophageal varicosities (varices)
Phlebitis, phlebothrombisis, arteritis

Conditions on or under the Skin
Acute neuritis
Frostbite
Any local contagious condition
Any local irritable skin condition
Any open wound or sore
Recent burns or scars
Abscesses
Severe gout
Hematoma
Ringworm
Cysts or foreign bodies
Scabies
Cellulitis (or the erysipelas that form)
Baker's cyst

Joints
Acute inflammatory arthrides (rheumatoid
  arthritis, systemic lupus erythematosis,
  ankylosing spondylitis)
Bursitis
Acute dislocation

Other Medical Conditions
Septic conditions
24–48 hours post-anti-inflammatory injection
site and immediate vicinity

RELATIVE
CONTRAINDICATIONS

Bones and Joints
Inflammatory arthrides (chronic phase)
Osteoporosis
Osteomalacia
Tuberculosis

Cancer
Any cancerous condition requires coordination
with other therapies.

Chronic Organ Diseases
Chronic congestive heart failure
Chronic kidney or liver disease
Chronic obstructive pulmonary disease
(COPD) (e.g. emphysema)
Diabetes (moderately severe)
Post-CVA
Post-MI

Circulatory Disorders
Hypertension
Diagnosed atherosclerosis
Anemia: sickle cell, hemorrhagic, hemolytic,
polycythemic, leukemic, or secondary

Drugs and Alcohol
Anti-inflammatories
Muscle relaxants
Anticoagulants
Analgesics
Any drug that alters sensation; muscle tone;
standard reflex reactions; personality; or
cardiovascular, kidney, or liver function
Alcohol
Narcotics or recreational drugs
Drug withdrawal

Neurologically Spastic or Rigid Conditions
Multiple sclerosis
Parkinson's disease

Cerebral palsy
Epilepsy
Signs such as numbness and weakness need
neurological referral

Other Medical Conditions
Immunosuppression
Coma
Major or abdominal surgery
Recent head injury

RELATIVE LOCAL
CONTRAINDICATIONS

Conditions on or under the skin
Contusions
Minor surgery
Trigeminal neuralgia
Neuritis

Bones and Joints
Acute disk herniation
Chronic arthritic conditions
Current or recent fracture
Joint instability or hypermobility

Circulatory Conditions
Mild to moderate aortic aneurism
Any chronic thrombosis
Portal hypertension
Hemorrhagic disorders and varicose veins

Internal Organs
Chronic abdominal / digestive disorders
Chronic diarrhea
Chronic constipation
Kidney infection or stones
Mastitis
Pelvic inflammatory disease
Ovarian cysts

Pregnancy
Lower abdomen
Yin legs
Points (Sp6, Sp8, St17, St25, St36, LI4,
Gb21, Li3, Bl60)
Recent abortion, miscarriage, or stillbirth
Recent delivery (vaginal or cesarean section)

Other Medical Conditions

Any acute inflammatory condition
Endometriosis
Flaccid paralysis or paresis
Hernia
Pitting edema

WARNINGS

General

Extreme client fatigue
Within one-half hour of eating
An undiagnosed condition
Pain of unknown cause
Sudden weight loss or gain for unknown reason
A frequent or persistent low-grade or
    intermittent fever
Night sweats
Sudden change in appetite for unknown reason
Undiagnosed lump or swelling

Personal

Practicing beyond your scope or training
When extremely off-centered
When extremely fatigued

Prosthetic Appliances

Pins and staples
Artificial joints

Client Allergies

Oils, creams, lotions, and liniments
Perfumes and scents
Cleaning chemicals

POTENTIAL ENDANGERMENT SITES

Nerves, arteries, veins, and lymph nodes as well as some of the more delicate organs can be harmed by excessive or extended pressure when these target areas lie on or close to the surface of the body. Great care must be taken when treating these areas.

Axilla (armpit)

Brachial plexus (lateral, medial, and posterior cords)

Axillary artery
Axillary vein
Axillary nerve
Lymph nodes

Medial Brachium (inner, upper arm between biceps and triceps)

Ulnar nerve
Median nerve
Musculocutaneous nerve
Brachial artery
Basilic vein

Additional considerations: In some people the radial nerve passes through the axilla and down the posterior side of the arm. In others it is found superior to the supraspinous fossa and then on the posterior aspect of the arm. The cephalic vein passes along the medial border of the deltoid and the lateral edge of the biceps.

Ulnar Notch ("funny bone")

The ulnar nerve is exposed when the arm is partially flexed.

Cubital Area (anterior elbow)

Median nerve
Radial artery
Ulnar artery
Median cubital vein

Femoral Triangle (groin/anterior hip— the area defined by the sartorius, adductor longus, and the inguinal ligament)

Lymph nodes
Femoral nerves
Femoral artery
Femoral vein
Great saphenous vein

Popliteal fossa (posterior knee— outlined by the hamstrings above and the gastrocnemius below)

Tibial nerve
Peroneal nerve
Popliteal artery
Popliteal nerve

Neck

Posterior neck

The occipital nerve is exposed at the base of the occiput when the head is hyperextended.

Anterior triangle (outlined by the trachea, sternocleidomastoid, and mandible)

Carotid artery

Internal jugular vein

Trachea

Vagus nerve

Lymph nodes

Posterior triangle (outlined by the clavicle, sternocleidomastoid, and transverse processes of the cervical spine)

Brachial plexus

Subclavian artery

Subclavian vein

External jugular vein

Lymph nodes

Notch posterior to the ramus of the mandible

Facial nerve

Trigeminal nerve

Styloid process

Coccyx (inferior tip of the spine)

Can be injured by too much pressure applied in a superior or posterior direction.

MEI GEN REACTION:
A HEALING CRISIS

THE WASTE AND TOXIC RESIDUE that the body has been unable to eliminate from the system progressively increases with age. These materials take the form of a crystalline coating that fills all the interstitial spaces of the body. Comprised of organic protein metabolites, by-products of muscular activity, or cellular detritus, much of this material coats the fascial sheaths surrounding the musculature of the body.[1] In large measure, this process accounts for the increasing density and decreasing pliability of aging tissues. The toxic degeneration of the tissues involved is also responsible for decreased sensitivity and responsiveness. Because the toxic buildup is a slow and gradual process, your client is not normally aware of this condition.

Digital compression—the principal technique of BodyWork Shiatsu—is uniquely effective in remobilizing this metabolic detritus. Deep compressions mechanically break these encrustations loose from their tissue beds, freeing them for transport by the lymphatic fluid transport system, the activity of which has been enhanced by the Body-Work Shiatsu treatment.

The sudden appearance of large quantities of toxic materials can severely stress the detoxification systems of the body. The mobilized materials are precisely those that the body has difficulty eliminating. Rapid systemic detoxification often brings, within twenty-four hours, the flulike symptoms of autointoxication: muscle soreness, aching joints, nausea, headache, depression, and so forth. In Oriental bodywork this reaction by the body is called a *mei gen* (or *menken*) reaction.[2] Although an acute detoxification reaction is ultimately beneficial, cleansing the body of years of accumulated toxins in a short period of time is very stressful. It is much more gentle to the client, and equally effective, to allow the elimination process to span several sessions.

The treatment of choice for a toxic client is preventive in nature—don't work too long or too deep in the first few sessions. It is also helpful to warn first-time clients of the possibility of a mei gen reaction, especially if you perceive them to be overly toxic. It's important that your client understand the nature of a healing crisis and work with the process instead of becoming frightened and thinking that you have done something "wrong" to make him or her sick. If you prepare your clients properly for the possibility of this reaction, and sensibly guide them through the appropriate detoxification procedures outlined below, you will be well on the road to establishing BodyWork Shiatsu, in their minds, as the potent therapeutic technique that it truly is.

As a precautionary measure, you should recommend that your clients drink one eight-ounce glass of water for every twenty pounds of body mass on the day of treatment and the following day. This will facilitate kidney filtration of the circulatory system. This is actually the amount of water a body needs every day in order to keep the tissues properly hydrated.[3] These requirements vary with activity level and climate. People who perspire heavily need more water. Advise those clients who are obviously very toxic to increase this fluid requirement by 25 percent for the thirty-six hours following each treatment.

EPSOM SALT BATH

Note: This procedure is contraindicated for clients with very high or very low blood pressure; with heart conditions or extreme circulatory problems; or for those who have been medically advised to avoid hot baths or who find hot baths too uncomfortable.

To prevent a mei gen reaction, to enhance and complete the relaxing qualities of your treatment, and to insure a good night's sleep, a very hot, highly concentrated Epsom salt bath should be recommended after every session. Since the toxic material that has been released from the tissues is floating in the superficial interstitial fluid, much of it can be pulled out of the body through the skin. If not eliminated, the tissues will reabsorb these irritating toxins within six to ten hours of their mobilization, in order to get them out of systemic circulation. The hot bath should be taken as soon after treatment as is feasible. Depending on the client's level of toxicity, twelve to sixteen pounds of salt should be used after the first treatment and eight to twelve pounds after each subsequent session.

Hot water causes the pores of the skin to open; Epsom salt (magnesium sulfate), a smooth-muscle relaxant, causes them to open further. The very high concentration of salt in the tub makes the bathwater denser than the interstitial fluid circulating in the body. This creates an osmotic pump effect, pulling the toxin-laden fluids out of the body through the skin by osmotic pressure. Because of the profuse perspiration provoked by this procedure, body fluid should be replenished by drinking eight to ten ounces of cool (not cold) water at the end the bath. For those who do not tolerate hot water well, an ice pack placed on the head during the bath will lower the temperature of the cerebral circulation and enable them to perform the procedure comfortably. The bath should last for 20 minutes or to tolerance.

The bath should immediately be followed by the coldest shower the client can tolerate. This will enhance systemic circulation by contrast rebound effect[4] and clean the skin of toxic residue. The shower must be long enough to close the pores and stop perspiration, which otherwise may continue for several hours, but not so long as to chill your client. Usually 30 to 45 seconds is enough, although longer is fine for clients who enjoy the cold water. A very cold climate, Cold internal conditions, or an aversion to cold water preclude the use of this technique.

Should your client call the day after treatment to report a mei gen reaction, you must be calm and reaffirm the beneficial nature of the healing crisis. The entire Epsom salt bath procedure should be repeated (usually the client will not have taken the bath after treatment as instructed). Suggest that the client receive a professional colonic irrigation or perform a high insertion enema to cleanse the colon of the waste eliminated by the digestive organs following the treatment.

HIGH INSERTION ENEMA

To perform the enema, a high-insertion colon tube—available at good drugstores and at surgical supply houses—should be attached to the end of the insert tip of the enema apparatus. The colon tube is inserted eight to ten inches into the colon, by way of the anus. Insertion to this depth allows the enema to bypass the pressure-receptive cells in the sigmoid colon. It thus eliminates the reflex opening of the internal anal sphincter, allowing the fluid to enter comfortably.

The enema is performed in three stages. The first insertion uses three cups of tepid (body temperature) water, which is immediately eliminated, to cleanse the sigmoid colon. The second insertion, also eliminated immediately, uses five cups of water to cleanse the descending colon. The third insertion, which uses seven cups of water to reach the transverse and ascending colon, should be retained

for fifteen minutes, if possible. During this time lie for five minutes on the right side, five minutes on your back (while performing circular kneading on the colon, clockwise from ileocecum to sigmoid), and five minutes on the left side. For the third insertion use tepid water with the strained juice of a freshly squeezed lemon. This will maximize mucosal discharge from the colon wall and increase peristaltic action, aiding in elimination.

Assume a supine position with the head resting on a pillow, the knees bent and the heels drawn up toward the buttocks. The enema apparatus should be hooked on a hanger and hung on a towel rack or shower curtain rod to let gravity produce insertion pressure. The rate of flow is controlled by pinching the tube open and closed. The secret of easeful insertion is to relax the abdomen and breathe deeply, thereby relaxing the colon and allowing it to expand to accommodate the insert. The entire procedure takes around forty-five minutes.

Give your client a very gentle, full-body treatment as soon as possible after this colon cleanse. This will relieve muscular soreness, stimulate vital energy circulation, and enable the two of you to reestablish positive contact. Above all, be clear and firm regarding the beneficial nature of a healing crisis. Be very reassuring about how much better your client will feel when the reaction runs its course. It's really true.

APPENDIX 3

A BIO-ELECTROMAGNETIC THEORY OF THE MERIDIANS AND ACUPOINTS

CONTRARY TO THE ASSUMPTIONS of modern Western science, many of the ancient great cultures were neither prescientific nor pretechnological; they were, rather, premechanical. Their science was of the energy body and the mind. Not locked in to the belief in the separation of energy from matter, of mind from body, they also pursued rigorous scientific explorations into the nature of reality. The goal of these inquiries, identical to the goal of our scientific culture, was to describe one unified theory of reality that would serve to relieve the suffering of humankind.

This basic drive of the human mind has not changed in all of the thousands of years of our evolutionary growth as a species. The ultimate nature of scientific inquiry, identical to the fundamental inquiry of the spiritual quest, is, and always has been, how to understand reality so that we can make life easier and more fulfilling. Whether we describe reality as Dao, Brahman, or God, this basic human impulse is to try to comprehend the nature of the universe in order to find the meaning and purpose of life and to put an end to suffering.

Science may be defined as "Knowledge acquired by careful observation, by deduction of the laws which govern changes and conditions, and by testing these deductions by experiment using methods based upon well-established facts and obeying well-established laws."[1] The Western scientific effort to affect and control matter, for example, has proceeded from deductions based on careful observation of the nature of the atom, to laws about that nature, to technological applications that demonstrate the validity of the laws we have postulated.

The ancient Oriental scientist-philosophers pursued the same quest using the technology of mind rather than the technology of matter. They used the concentrated mind as the instrument of observation. Their exploration led them from the subtlest level of awareness achievable, the utter stillness of the Self, outward toward the grossest manifestation of the bodymind in the phenomenal world. That exploration resulted in scientific laws regarding reality that are replicable by anyone who utilizes the appropriate technology. After roughly three hundred years of scientific inquiry, our culture is just beginning to apply its technology successfully to these subtle energetic and mental realms that the ancients explored thousands of years ago.

The basis for the hypothesis I am proposing to describe the etymology and function of the regular meridians and the Extraordinary Vessels comes from the work of one of the greatest scientists of the twentieth century, Dr. Robert O. Becker. An orthopedic surgeon beginning his research into the causes of nonunion fractures in 1958, Dr. Becker's eclectic genius and endless curiosity led him to explore an incredible range of subjects dealing with bio-electromagnetism in the human body. Integrating information from a truly awesome range of scientific disciplines, Dr. Becker postulated the dual nervous system (DNS) hypothesis in 1976.

Dr. Becker postulated that the DNS consists of a primitive analog, direct-current (DC) component that appeared early in evolution, and a more sophisticated digital, nerve-impulse component of more recent origin. He theorized that our bodies have an intricate and multilayered self-regulating feedback arrangement made up of a high-speed digital-impulse network operating through the nervous system, which directly controls all physiological end-organs (the expanded end of nerve fibers in peripheral structures that allow the signals of the autonomic and central nervous systems to control all of the sensorimotor and organ tissues of the body), and a more primitive DC analog control system operating through the perineural network of myelin sheaths, Schwann cells, and neuroglial cells which cover and support every part of the nervous system. He posited that this analog portion of the DNS is responsible for control of such poorly understood mental functions as regulating changes in consciousness and the perception of pain. He also

suggested that it acts as an electrical bias control for the neural network, stabilizing the direction, speed, and frequency of the nerve impulses throughout the body. Moreover, he felt that the analog system may well prove to be a bridge to understanding such other human functions as memory and emotion and even creative inspiration. [2]

Expanding on Dr. Becker's dual nervous system (DNS) hypothesis, I conjecture that, in addition to the perineural relationship with the neurons of the central and autonomic nervous systems, it is the regular meridians that are used by the brain/mind to maintain analogue awareness and control of the functioning of all of the major organ systems of the body. I also postulate that the Extraordinary Vessel system performs a similar function in controlling both embryological development and gross structural balance. These complex networks act as part of the information and control system of the brain/mind, interacting with and regulating the digital neurological communication networks to form the dual autonomic and central nervous systems.

Following Dr. Becker, I postulate that the basic DC current generated by the limbic system of the brain, which uses the perineural network to form the analog complement to the digital functions of the neurons, additionally forms a secondary set of analog connections via the autonomic nervous system with the developing internal organs. I believe that the basic DC current that Dr. Becker has discovered flowing along the perineural network thus represents an analogous phenomenon to that which the Chinese called the meridian system. Partially utilizing the perineural portion of the DNS and partially following very complex courses of superficial and deep pathways that follow various tissue phase boundaries, this system maintains the analog portion of communication between the internal organs and the brain/mind.

According to TCM theory, the pathway system begins to form at conception, although the regular meridians don't become active until birth. The Extraordinary Vessels begin to form with the dividing ovum and control the actual structural unfolding of the developing fetus. According to the British mathematician John Evens, the energy for these transformations is inherent in the DNA molecule itself.[3] Jing from the Kidneys of the parents, derived from their Prenatal Qi, flows through these developing Extraordinary Vessels guiding embryological development. According to Dr. Yoshio Manaka, the Extraordinary Vessels represent the control mechanism that guides the initial stages of embryogenesis. It is at this time when gross structure and the earliest differentiations of the embryo into ectodermal, mesodermal, and endodermal tissues take place. Manaka proposes that the first division of the ovum into two cells represents the formation of the Ren Mai–Du Mai pair of Extraordinary Vessels, which separate the front and back of the body into left and right halves and exert fundamental control of the Yin and Yang functions of the body. He further postulates that the second division into four cells represents the formation of the Dai Mai Vessel, separating top from bottom (fig. A.1).[4]

Departing from Dr. Manaka, I speculate that the first division of the fertilized ovum into two cells is the concrete manifestation of the Oriental cosmological division of the One into the Two, the first separation of Yin and Yang, prior to the formation of the Extraordinary Vessels. Embryologically, the first division of the fertilized zygote, which occurs along the polar axis of the ovum, splits the original cell into two cells called blastomeres. These two cells are called the epiblast and the hypoblast. While both of these cells rapidly divide over and over within the zona pellucida, the original membrane of the fertilized zygote, the size of the cell mass is not increased. This stage, called

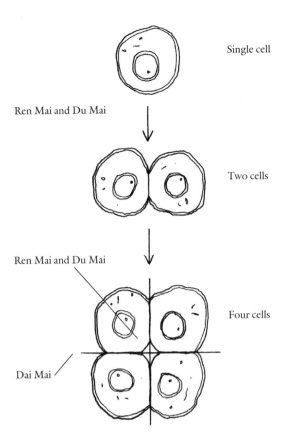

Single cell

Ren Mai and Du Mai

Two cells

Ren Mai and Du Mai

Four cells

Dai Mai

Fig. A.1. Formation of the Ren Mai, Du Mai, and Dai Mai from the Ovum

cleavage, marks the beginning of the process of differentiation. The epiblast splits into the rudiments of the Yang, membranous covering of the developing fetus, called the trophectoderm. This cell layer ultimately develops into the chorion, the covering that connects the fetus to the mother's uterus. The divisions of the hypoblast, the second blastomere, takes place within the trophectoderm, initially filling it, and forming the inner cell mass that ultimately differentiates into the fetus itself, which is Yin relative to the covering membrane. This represents the first differentiation into Yin and Yang.

After the first differentiation into epiblast and hypoblast, the cleavage period results in the formation of the morula (mulberry) (fig. A.2). This is a solid mass of undifferentiated hypoblastic cells covered by a layer of undifferentiated epiblastic cells.

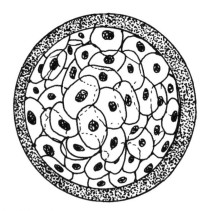

Fig. A.2. Morula

This process, which takes about five days, marks the movement of the zygote through the fallopian tube to the uterus.

As the morula passes into the uterus, the dense clustering of hypoblastic cells within the trophectoderm begins to dissolve, leaving an inner cell mass of hypoblastic cells at one portion of the trophectoderm, surrounded by a fluid-filled space called the blastocoel. Now called a blastocyst, the zygote implants into the endometrial lining of the uterine wall (fig. A.3). The inner cell mass, called the embryonal pole, is oriented directly toward the uterine wall.

About the sixth day after fertilization an amazing transformation occurs. It is this that I believe marks the initial formation of the Ren Mai and Du Mai (Conception and Governor Vessels). The undifferentiated hypoblast, the inner cell mass, splits into a bilaminar plate formed of two entirely different types of cell that will eventually form all of the ectodermal and endodermal tissues of the body. The ectoderm will ultimately differentiate into the entire nervous system and the epidermis, the most Yang parts of the body, controlled by the Du Mai, which passes up the posterior midline overlying the developing neural canal. The endoderm will differentiate into the digestive tube and the glands and organs that open into it as well as the respiratory organs, the most Yin portions of the body, controlled by the Ren Mai that passes up the ventral midline directly over the earliest stages of the developing gut (fig. A.4).

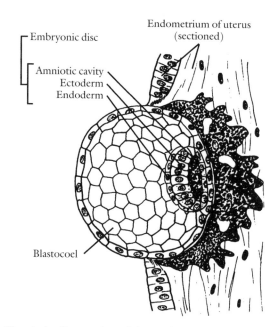

Fig. A.4. Formation of the Embryonic Disc

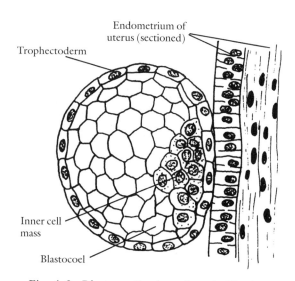

Fig. A.3. Blastocyst Implanted on the Uterine Endometrium

During the second week of embryological development, called gastrulation, the initial movements toward the formation of the neurological and digestive tubes begin to take place. The portion of the inner cell mass that has differentiated into ectodermal tissue and is in contact with the chorion splits so that a layer of ectoderm remains in contact with the chorion while the main mass of ectodermal tissue moves further into the blastocoel with the rest of the embryonic disk. This allows a cavity within the ectoderm, called the amniotic cavity, to begin to form above the developing embryo. Ultimately the entire fetus will develop within this protective sack. The bottom portion of the embryonic disk, meanwhile, has differentiated into the endodermal layer (fig. A.5).

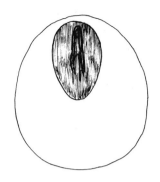

Fig. A.6. *Primitive Streak of a Seven-day Rabbit Embryo*

germ layer, begins to form. The ectoderm on either side of the primitive streak begins to proliferate and thicken at the same time that the underlying endodermal cells also begin to proliferate, becoming indistinguishable from the overlying ectoderm and raising up to form the primitive groove. These ridges form plates, the laminae dorsales, which converge to form the neural canal in the ectoderm. Just below this, above the endoderm, a row of mesodermic cells form into the notochord, which eventually differentiates into the spinal column (fig. A.7).

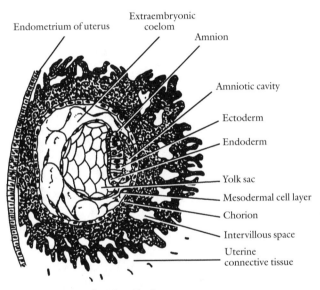

Fig. A.5. *Twelve-day Embryo*

Labels: Endometrium of uterus · Extraembryonic coelom · Amnion · Amniotic cavity · Ectoderm · Endoderm · Yolk sac · Mesodermal cell layer · Chorion · Intervillous space · Uterine connective tissue

By the twelfth day the endodermal layer has proliferated and spread downward to form the yolk sac. The entire bilaminar plate has taken the form of an oval disk with the broader end in contact with the trophectoderm and the pointed end oriented into the blastocoel. Now the primitive streak begins to form in the ectoderm along the embryonic axis, directly over the emerging midline of the developing embryo (fig. A.6).

By the fourteenth day the mesoderm, the third

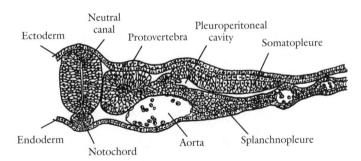

Fig. A.7. *Neural Canal and Notochord*

Labels: Ectoderm · Neutral canal · Protovertebra · Pleuroperitoneal cavity · Somatopleure · Endoderm · Notochord · Aorta · Splanchnopleure

From the lateral sides of the dorsal laminae and partly derived from both ectoderm and endoderm, mesodermic cells pour out, filling the space that forms between the ectoderm and endoderm with a longitudinal ridge of mesodermal tissue that I believe represents the initial formation of the Chong Mai (Penetrating Vessel). These mesodermal ridges thicken and grow, forming the aorta and vena cava as well as the paraxial mesoblasts, which differentiate over time into two rows of protovertebrae or mesoblastic somites. These, in turn, split to form the vertebral column as well as the muscles, fascia, and skin of the back. At the edges of the protovertebrae the lateral mesoblast splits to form the pleuro-peritoneal cavity, with the upper layer joining the ectoderm to form the somatopleure (the body wall) and the skin. The lower layer joins the endoderm to form the splanchnopleure, the alimentary canal. Thus, from an embryological point of view, the Du Mai, Ren Mai, and Chong Mai all originate from the three fundamental tissue types differentiating from the primitive streak at the core of the body.

These three Extraordinary Vessels share a profound and intimate relationship in Chinese medical theory. The Du Mai, Ren Mai, and Chong Mai all originate in the central energetic field of the body, the "small abdomen" or "moving Qi between the Kidneys." Li Shi Zhen said of this relationship: "The Triple Heater is the function of Ming Men. The Ren Mai and Du Mai make contact together at the Chong Mai."[5] The Ren and Du Mai are not separate pathways, but rather the first separation of Yin and Yang at the energetic level. They originate in the root of the Chong Mai. The Chong Mai represents the abdominal blood vessels, the course of the deep blood circulation, hence its designation as the "ocean of the twelve meridians, the five Yin and six Yang Organs, and the ocean of the Blood." The relationship between autonomic function and arterial circulation is clear. Wang Bing, one of the most famous commentators on the *Su Wen*, said: "This is why we can say that the Du Mai, Ren Mai, and Chong Mai have different names but are all the same."[6]

By the end of the third week the cephalic and caudal ends of the embryo begin to curve toward one another, and the sides of the embryonic plate wrap ventrally inward to enclose the enteron (embryonic alimentary canal). The entire embryo takes on a canoe-shaped form, pinching off the fetus proper from the yolk sac. I believe the formation of this limiting sulcus, which in time becomes the umbilicus, indicates the activation of the Dai Mai (Belt Vessel) and marks the beginning of the cylindrical shape of the human organism (fig. A.8).

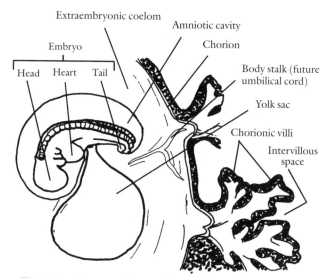

Fig. A.8. Enteron (Canoe Shape)

Thus, very early in embryonic development, three parallel structures form along the central polar axis directly on the midline. The neural tube, formed from the ectoderm and the most dorsal of these structures, is directly related to the Du Mai. The gut tube—originally a vertical canal formed from the endoderm along the ventral midline—is related to the Ren Mai (fig. A.9). The notochord and aorta, formed from the emerging mesoderm directly between the neural and gut tubes, represents the emergent Chong Mai.[7] Following Manaka, I believe that the anterior, midline, and poste-

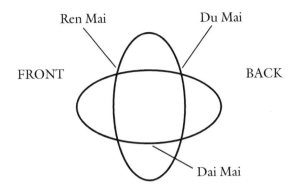

Fig. A.9. The Ren Mai, Du Mai, and Dai Mai Define a Cylinder

rior orientation of these physical structures is responsible for the Great Energy meridian relationships. Thus the Yang Ming–Tai Yin meridians (Stomach/Large Intestine and Lung/Spleen) are on the ventral surface of the body, the Tai Yang–Shao Yin meridians (Bladder/Small Intestine and Kidney/Heart) lie on the dorsal surface, and the Shao Yang–Jue Yin meridians (Gallbladder/Triple Heater and Liver/Heart Envelope) are on the midline.

By the end of the fourth week of development the limb buds begin to form from a thickening at the lateral edge of the somatopleure (body wall). I believe this marks the emergence of the Yin and Yang Wei Mai and Qiao Mai (Linking and Heel Vessels), which control the raising and lowering of both Yin Qi and Yang Qi in the body and are also intimately connected to the formation of the courses of the regular meridians on the limbs. I believe that the emergence of the Wei Mai and Qiao Mai are the root cause of the electrical gradients that lead the growing nerve fibers to innervate the mesenchymal tissues of the limb buds, causing them to differentiate into all of the different tissues of the limbs.[8] Each of the Wei and Qiao Mai is coupled with one of the primary, core Extraordinary Vessels in a therapeutic pairing, as described in the section on Extraordi-

nary Vessels, and is also involved in the structural division of the body into Octants.

Dr. Yoshio Manaka developed this topologic approach to the control of the structural development of the body based on his etymological research into the original meanings of the ideograms classically used to describe the Extraordinary Vessels.[9] The Du Mai ascends the posterior midline, the Ren Mai ascends the anterior midline, and the Dai Mai circles the waist (fig. A.10). This produces a relatively equal sectioning of the fetus along Yin-Yang lines. Coining the term *octants,* he further points out that the Triple Heater and Gallbladder meridians divide the front and back aspects of the Yang portion of the body, and the Heart Envelope and Spleen meridians divide the midline of the Yin portion. The Yin and Yang Wei Mai have their Master Points on the Heart Envelope and Triple Heater meridians respectively. Treatment points for the Chong and Dai Mai lie on the Spleen and Gallbladder meridians. The Yin and Yang Qiao Mai have Master Points on the Kidney and Bladder meridians, proximate to the Ren Mai and Du Mai channels, completing this structural pattern.[10]

I speculate that secondary to the formation of the Extraordinary Vessels and the DNS—but building on it—is the formation of the Regular

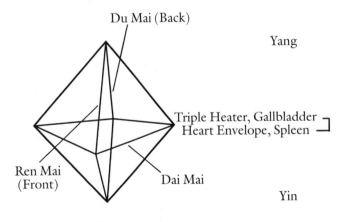

Fig. A.10. Manaka's Octants

Meridian system. As the internal organs of the fetus begin developing, the superficial and deep courses of the regular meridians also begin to form, following the embryological course of the developing organs and the autonomic nerves that innervate them. I speculate that they are directed on the arms and legs by the Wei Mai and Qiao Mai as they guide limb-bud formation. Chinese medicine points out that the meridians that develop on the arms either represent the most Yang Organ/Elements of Fire and Metal and lie in the Upper Heater or are Element-related to the Yin Organs that do. The pathways of the legs represent the more Yin Elements—Earth, Water, and Wood—and occupy the Middle and Lower Heaters. I speculate that the creation of the meridians represents the emergence of the superficial analog portion of the dual autonomic nervous system (DANS) that manifests with the autonomic nerves that control the internal organs.

On the limbs the meridians trace various nerve routes, although not necessarily contiguous ones. On the torso they follow autonomic nerve pathways or the tissue phase boundaries of the various planes of fascia that they passed through during embryological development.[11] Pathways may also pass along the major circulatory vessels. The common thread among all of these different physical pathways is that each of them has a clear-cut tissue-phase boundary that can support direct current electrical transmission.[12] Although nerves themselves are not electrically contiguous with each other, the neuroglial and perineural tissues surrounding and supporting them do form a physically continuous syncytium that is capable of direct current transmission.[13] (A syncytium is a group of cells in which the protoplasm of one cell is continuous with that of adjoining cells, such as the mesenchyme cells of the embryo or the support cells of the neurons). This allows a continuous pathway for the transmission of DC signals.

I theorize that communication of information through the meridians is accomplished by a process I call *electromembranous communication*. This refers to the method of information transfer utilizing the natural direct current electrical signals produced by the limbic system of the brain, as well as modulations of that basic current and the electromagnetic fields thereby generated, and transmitted along the course of the various superficial and deep tissue phase-boundaries of the body that comprise the analog meridian system in order to maintain instantaneous, bidirectional communication between all parts of the body and the brain/mind. The brain/mind is able to affect change by direct electrical or magnetic stimulation or sedation of selected target end-organs, while the body can equally and reciprocally affect changes in the brain/mind through the same electromagnetic mechanisms.

We may conceptualize the communication of this analog portion of the dual analog-digital brain/mind control system as similar to radio wave transmissions. The fundamental action of a radio transmitter is the generation of a basic carrier wave, receivable by every radio that is tuned to the proper frequency. This wave does not carry information on its own, but rather establishes basic communication between the transmitter and the radio. In order for the carrier wave to transmit specific information it must be modulated. In our modern radio transmission technology this is done by modulating the amplitude or size of the wave (AM radio) or by modulating the frequency or rate of vibration of the wave (FM radio).

In a similar fashion, I postulate that brain/mind is in constant, bidirectional communication with all of the end-organs of the body through the dual nervous system and that the various manipulations of Oriental medicine alter the fundamental signal passing through the analog meridian system in such a way as to recreate balance, when it has been disturbed, in either the brain/mind or the target end-organs. The internal Organs and their functions, as identified by Chinese medical theory, are the principal end-organs of this system. The signals are unique to each of the Organ/meridians in a fashion that identifies it unmistakably to the brain/mind. Through this mechanism extremely fine distinctions between the normal, excess, or deficient functioning of each Organ/system can be constantly monitored and controlled by the brain/mind.[14] The functional state of each Organ/system is reflected on the surface of the body and can therefore by affected by the various techniques of Oriental medicine.

Research by Dr. Becker has shown that collagen, a basic component of the connective tissue that holds every part of the human body together, is a piezoelectric colloidal protein. This means that pressure applied to any collaginous tissue generates an electrical discharge.[15] I believe these minute electrical signals, which may only be on the order of millionths or billionths of an ampere, can have a significant physiological effect when traveling along the electrically facilitated pathway system. Research shows that signals of such tiny electrical magnitude may be within the range of physiological effectiveness.[16] This would mean that minute levels of stimulation could have profound biological effects when applied at exactly the proper location, with appropriate skill.

Along the superficial course of these meridians the skin and superficial fascia exhibit pathways of diminished resistance to the passage of electromagnetic energy, which carries specific information about each of the Organ/functions. Compared to normal tissue, the meridians provide a distinct reduction of resistance to electrical transmission.[17] I believe this phenomena is created by induction from the underlying meridian current passing along the specific phase boundary of each pathway. The sensitivity and speed of this analog component, balanced by the complexity and much slower speed of neural communication, allows for the ability of the brain/mind to read and respond to imbalances and blockages in the meridian network.[18] These superficial facilitated pathways are the focus of the Sphere of Heaven meridian-targeted manipulations.

I believe that treatment of the acupoints initiate their effects in two ways. The most immediate effects are initiated through the same direct current electromembranous signals used by the analog meridian system to affect their target end-organs. This effect takes place through the perineural covering of the nerves. Secondly, I conjecture that effects are also generated by a process I call *neuroionic communication*. This refers to the method of information transfer that uses direct current electrical signals or the electromagnetic fields they generate to modulate the ionic resting or action potential of the neurons or the polarity of their syncytia, in order to control their rate of firing, the intensity of that activity, or the threshold of stimulation necessary in order to activate them, as the primary mechanism for affecting change in the target end-organs. By controlling the level of stimulus necessary to affect communication through the various axons of the nervous system you control the information they communicate, modulating it as appropriate. This allows for the selective stimulation or sedation of specific target end-organs by the acupoint-directed techniques of Oriental medicine.

Because of the neurological basis of this feedback mechanism, changes created with this system take longer than the analog meridian system does to affect their target areas. This is because the mode of communication is inherently slower than electromembranous communication, which takes place at the speed with which direct currents can travel along the meridians. Neuroionic information is transmitted by the ion exchange method of all neural transmission, and such impulses travel between 1½ and 400 feet per second, depending on the thickness and myelinization of the involved nerves.[19] However, because of the direct effect of neuroionic communication on the central and autonomic nervous systems, these effects are relatively more profound than those created electromembranously through the analog meridian system.

It has also been postulated by Dr. Becker that some of the acupoints act as step-up transformers, maintaining the level of direct-current electricity being transmitted through the pathways against the electrical resistance of the tissues. It has long been recognized that only 70 percent of the body's acupoints are always palpable. Thirty percent of the points only become active when there is an imbalance present.[20] Some of these acupoints may be activated in a reflexive response to internal imbalances, but some might well play a role as electrical transformers, maintaining signal amplitude along the lines of direct-current communication. Although the current draining effects of the conducting medium may be ameliorated by biological superconduction,[21] it seems possible that the point and pathway communication systems incorporate some sort of alternative mechanism for maintaining the amplitude of signals within the network.

NOTES

指圧

CHAPTER 1

1. S. Masunaga with W. Ohashi, *Zen Shiatsu* (Tokyo: Japan Press, 1977).

2. Ibid. Also H. Lee and G. Whincup, *Chinese Massage Therapy: A Handbook of Therapeutic Massage* (Boulder, Colo.: 1983); K. Serizawa, *Tsubo: Vital Points for Oriental Therapy* (Tokyo: Japan Publishers, 1976); and T. Namikoshi, *The Complete Book of Shiatsu* (Tokyo: Japan Publishers, 1981).

3. In the summer of 1989 leaders of the American Shiatsu Association, the Midwest Shiatsu Association, the Shiatsu/Anma Practitioners Association of California, and the Jin Shin Do Foundation, as well as leading educators and school owners from across the United States, met for two consecutive weekends, first in Oak Park, Illinois, for the first International Federation of the Natural Healing Arts, and one week later in Kerhonset, New York, for the 4th annual American Shiatsu Association convention. After exhaustive discussion, all representatives agreed to merge the existing regional Oriental bodywork associations into one national association.

4. C. Dubitsky, et al. "Three Paradigms, Five Approaches." *Massage Therapy Journal* (Summer 1991).

5. S. Masunaga with W. Ohashi, *Zen Shiatsu*.

6. R. Lee and G. Whincup, *Chinese Massage Therapy*.

7. Serizawa, *Tsubo*.

8. This information about Waichi Sugiyama was given to me orally by Toshiko Phipps.

9. Junji Mizutani, "A Brief History." *Shiatsu Therapy of Ontario Newsletter* (September 1991).

10. According to Masunaga Sensei, this work was the prototype for the development of shiatsu. See note 5.

11. Toshiko Phipps translated this passage for me from a manuscript in her possession.

12. During the first International Shiatsu Summit in 1989, Toru Namikoshi, the son of Tokujiro Namikoshi, told me that the trigger point massage technique created by Dr. Janet Travell was based on information she recieved from Namikoshi during his first visit to the United States in 1953.

13. When the victorious American troops began repatriating GIs who had been interned in prisoner-of-war camps, the POWs told horror stories of being burned and stuck with needles when they got sick. Today we know that some of these practices were attempts to provide Oriental medical care to the sick GIs, but in the aftermath of the war they appeared to be a form of torture and resulted in General MacArthur outlawing the practices of acupuncture and moxibustion in Japan.

14. K. Matsumoto and S. Birch, *Hara Diagnosis: Reflections on the Sea* (Brookline, Mass.: Paradigm Publishers, 1988).

15. Moxibustion is the technique of applying heat to an acupoint, or pathway, by burning the dried, processed leaves of the mugwort *(Artemisia vulgaris)*. Moxa, or mogusa, as the herbal preparation is called, can be applied directly to the skin of an acu-

point, or indirectly by placing thin slices of different substances (such as ginger or garlic) between the moxa and the skin or by using "cigars" of rolled-up moxa near the skin. Moxa may also be applied by wrapping the herbal preparation around the handle of an inserted acupuncture needle and burning it. The herb itself has therapeutic properties, and the heat adds energy to the region or reflex point to which it is applied.

16. Please see my article "Three Paradigms, Five Approaches" in *Massage Therapy Journal*, Summer 1991, for a more comprehensive discussion of the general context of these three levels of practice throughout the massage and bodywork profession.

17. Ogawa Harukai, *Lao Tze and Chuag Tze, Dao De Jing* (Tokyo: Chuo Koran, 1978).

Chapter 2

1. F. Capra, *The Tao of Physics* (New York: Bantam, 1976).

2. Ogawa Harukai, *Lao Tze and Chuag Tze, Dao De Jing* (Tokyo: Chuo Koran, 1978).

3. A. Ellis, N. Wiseman, and K. Boss, *Fundamentals of Chinese Acupuncture* (Brookline, Mass.: 1988).

4. Ibid.

5. K. Matsumoto and S. Birch, *Five Elements and Ten Stems* (Brookline, Mass.: Paradigm Publications, 1983).

6. Ibid.

7. R. Becker and A. Marino, *Electromagnetism and Life* (Albany, N.Y.: State University of New York, 1982).

8. K. Nakagawa, "Magnetic Field Deficiency Syndrome and Magnetic Treatment." *Japan Medical Journal* 2745 (1976): December 4.

9. Ibid.

10. Becker and Marino, *Electromagnetism.*

11. Both the Greco-Roman and Aryan cultures differentiated the elements according to their structural qualities. Differentiating either four or five elements, these cultures divided the natural world into solid, liquid, gas, fire, and in some cases ether (or vacuum), thus marking the major distinct phases of manifestation in the sensory world.

12. The eight trigrams are combinations of three solid and/or broken lines representing all of the Yin or Yang qualities found in nature. The oldest depiction of these symbols has been found on bones used for divination during the Shang dynasty, 1500 B.C.E. In the I Jing, written approximately 1000 B.C.E., the author, King Wen, doubled up the trigrams to produce sixty-four hexagrams, which he used as symbols

for all of the possible changes described by his philosophical system. Although still best known as a system of fortune telling or divination, the I Jing is in reality a profound philosophical guide to the right actions of the Superior Man. See H. Wilhelm, *The I Ching,* Bollingen ed. xix (Princeton University Press, 1950).

13. Matsumoto and Birch, *Five Elements.*

14. Ibid.

15. Ibid.

16. Ibid.

17. Matsumoto and Birch, *Hara Diagnosis.*

18. T. Sohn and R. Sohn, *Amma Therapy: A Complete Textbook of Oriental Bodywork and Medical Principles* (Rochester, Vt.: Healing Arts Press, 1996).

19. Matsumoto and Birch, *Five Elements;* D. Connelly, *Traditional Acupuncture: The Law of the Five Elements* (Columbia, Md.: Centre for Traditional Acupuncture, 1979).

Chapter 3

1. G. Maciocia, *Foundations of Chinese Medicine* (Edinburgh: Churchill Livingstone, 1989).

2. Ibid.

3. The law of karma is a universal tenet in all Eastern spiritual traditions and was also recognized by the Catholic Church until the fourth century C.E. Briefly stated, the law of karma is a spiritual formulation of Newton's third law of motion: For every action there is an equal and opposite reaction. In human terms this means that, over the course of eternity, every action performed by an embodied being out of ignorance of the truth will cause a repercussion meant to point to that truth of which the being was ignorant. This is not a statement of the vindictiveness of the universe but rather of the "educational" nature of life, with the endless opportunity each moment affords us to awaken to the truth of reality.

4. Maciocia, *Foundations* .

5. Ibid.

6. Ibid.

7. Ibid.

8. Ellis, Wiseman, and Boss, *Fundamentals.*

9. Ibid.

10. Ibid.

11. Matsumoto and Birch, *Five Elements.*

12. Ibid.

13. Macioca, *Foundations.*

14. Ibid.

15. Ibid.

16. Ibid.

17. Ibid.

18. Ibid.
19. Ibid.
20. Ibid.
21. Ibid.
22. Ibid.
23. Ibid.
24. Ibid.
25. Ibid.
26. Ibid.
27. Ibid.
28. J. Ross, *Zang Fu: The Organ Systems of Traditional Chinese Medicine*, 2nd ed. (Edinburgh: Churchill Livingston, 1985).
29. Maciocia, *Foundations.*
30. Ibid.
31. Ibid.

CHAPTER 4

1. T. Kaptchuk, *The Web That Has No Weaver* (New York: Congdon and Weed, 1983).
2. Ibid.
3. Ellis, Wiseman, and Boss, *Fundamentals.*
4. Ibid.
5. K. Matsumoto and S. Birch, *Extraordinary Vessels* (Brookline, Mass.: Paradigm Publications, 1986).
6. Ibid.
7. Ibid.
8. Matsumoto and Birch, *Hara Diagnosis.*
9. D. Bohm, *Wholeness and the Implicate Order* (London: Ark Paperbacks, 1981).
10. Matsumoto and Birch, *Extraordinary Vessels.*
11. Ibid.
12. Dr. Y. Manaka, as quoted in Matsumoto and Birch, *Extraordinary Vessels.*
13. Matsumoto and Birch, *Extraordinary Vessels.*
14. See section on structure and function in chapter 6.
15. Y. Requena, *Terrains and Pathology in Acupuncture* (Brookline, Mass.: Paradigm Publishers, 1988).
16. Matsumoto and Birch, *Extraordinary Vessels.*

CHAPTER 5

1. Ellis, Wiseman, and Boss, *Fundamentals.*
2. Ibid.
3. Maciocia, *Foundations.*
4. In *Hara Diagnosis*, Matsumoto and Birch point out that the literal translation of the injurious emotion of the heart is "joy of overeating." This is certainly consistent with the modern findings of Western science.
5. See Kaptchuk's introduction to Ellis, Wiseman, and Boss, *Fundamentals of Chinese Medicine.*

6. Ibid.
7. Ellis, Wiseman, and Boss, *Fundamentals.*
8. Sun Chengnan, ed., *Chinese Bodywork: A Complete Manual of Chinese Therapeutic Massage* (Berkeley, Calif.: Pacific View Press, 1993).
9. This occurred during my clinical training with Dr. K. Nakamura in New York City in 1975–76.
10. Ellis, Wiseman, and Boss, *Fundamentals.*
11. Ibid.
12. Ibid.
13. Ibid.
14. Kaptchuk, *Web.*
15. Maciocia, *Foundations.*
16. Ibid.
17. Ibid.
18. Matsumoto and Birch, *Five Elements.*
19. In a few people, the radial artery is on the outside of the styloid process. This is a natural anatomical variation, not a pathological condition.
20. Maciocia, *Foundations.*
21. Kaptchuk, *Web.*
22. Requena, *Terrains.*
23. Ibid
24. Dr. T. Kaneko, course notes, 1978-79.
25. Matsumoto and Birch, *Hara Diagnosis.*
26. Maciocia, *Foundations.*
27. Ibid.

CHAPTER 6

1. Care must be taken to distinguish the "E" series of prostaglandins, which serve a humero-regulatory function for the female hormone system, from the pro-inflammatory "F" series. When the essential fatty acid metabolism, which underlies appropriate hormone function, is deranged, usually because of dietary indiscretion, hormone synthesis in the female system gets blocked at the metabolic step between linoleic and linolenic acid. This forms the basis of the use of evening primrose oil, which is very high in gamma-linolenic acid, a direct precursor of "E" series prostaglandins, to correct premenstrual hormonal imbalances. For more information on this subject see J. Graham, *Evening Primrose Oil* (Rochester, Vt.: Healing Arts Press, 1984).
2. D. Juhan, *Job's Body* (Barrytown, N.Y.: Station Hill Press, 1987).
3. S. Haldeman, *Modern Developments in the Principles and Practice of Chiropractic* (New York: Appleton-Century-Crofts, 1981).
4. I. Rolf, *Integration of Human Structures* (Santa Monica, Calif.: Landman Publishers, 1977).

5. Ibid.

6. J. Upledger and J. Vredevoogd, *Craniosacral Therapy* (Seattle: Eastland Press, 1983).

7. Ibid.

8. The liver, gallbladder, stomach, large intestine, small intestine, and bladder are directly palpable; the pancreas and kidneys are partially palpable; the heart, lungs, and spleen are manipulable through mobilization of the rib cage. See J. P. Barral and P. Mercier, *Visceral Manipulation* (Seattle: Eastland Press, 1988).

9. Masunaga, *Zen Shiatsu*.

10. See the discussion of stereotaxis in the section on structure and function.

11. H. Selye, *The Stress of Life* (New York: McGraw-Hill, 1976).

12. *The New Lexicon Webster's Dictionary of the English Language* (New York: Lexicon Press, 1984).

13. Ibid.

14. *Taber's Cyclopedic Medical Dictionary* (Philadelphia: Davis, 1981).

15. The three dimensions are the length, depth, and breadth of an object in space. The fourth dimension is time.

16. L. Chaitow, *Soft Tissue Manipulation* (Rochester, Vt.: Healing Arts Press, 1987); see also Rolf, *Integration*.

17. G. Tortora and N. Anagnostakos, *Principles of Anatomy and Physiology,* 4th ed. (New York: Harper and Row, 1984).

18. J. Evens, *Mind, Body and Electromagmetism* (Longmead, U.K.: Element Books, 1981).

19. Selye, *Stress of Life.*

20. Ibid.

21. E. and A. Green, *Beyond Biofeedback* (San Francisco: Delacourt Press, 1977).

22. Ibid.

23. Tortora and Anagnostakos, *Principles.*

24. B. Benjamin, *Listen To Your Pain* (New York: Penguin Books, 1984).

25. *Taber's Medical Dictionary.*

26. L. Jones, *Strain and Counterstrain* (Colorado Springs: American Academy of Osteopathy, 1981).

27. Ibid.

CHAPTER 7

1. *Taber's Medical Dictionary.*

2. Juhan, *Job's Body.*

3. For an in-depth discussion of subtle hygiene, see M. Chia, *Chi Nei Tsang* (Huntington, N.Y.: Healing Tao Books, 1990).

CHAPTER 8

1. The planes of the fascial sheaths within the body run in a generally longitudinal direction. There are three regions of transverse restriction—the thoracic inlet, the respiratory diaphragm, and the pelvic diaphragm. These horizontal restrictions limit and stabilize the top of the thorax, the abdomino-thoracic boundary, and the base of the torso. While necessary for the physical coherence of the torso, these regions are prone to restrictions that have far-reaching consequences. For a detailed discussion of these restrictions and their treatment, see Upledger and Vredevoogd, *Craniosacral Therapy.*

APPENDIX 2

1. Juhan, *Job's Body.*

2. Masunaga, *Zen Shiatsu.*

3. This information comes from private lessons given me by Toshiko Phipps.

4. The superficial capillary beds will have opened to about 75 percent of their capacity because of the wet heat. When immediately subjected to the cold water, they will snap shut, then reflexly open completely by contrast rebound effect. See F. Moor et al., *Manual of Hydrotherapy and Massage* (Mountain View, Calif.: Pacific Press, 1964).

APPENDIX 3

1. *New Lexicon Webster's.*

2. For a thorough and exciting history of this genius's work, as well as an account of his efforts to alert the American public to the hidden dangers of the effects of electromagnetic radiation, see R. Becker and G. Seldon, *The Body Electric: Electromagnetism and the Foundation of Life* (New York: William Morrow, 1985).

3. Evens, *Mind, Body and Electromagnetism.*

4. As quoted in Matsumoto and Birch, *Hara Diagnosis,* from an original paper entitled "Shinkyu no Riron to Kangaikata" handed out by Dr. Y. Manaka at his lectures.

5. Li Shi Zhen, *Qi Jing Ba Mai Kao,* as quoted in Matsumoto and Birch, *Extraordinary Vessels.*

6. Wang Bing, *Nei Jing Jie Po Sheng Li Xue,* as quoted in Matsumoto and Birch, *Extraordinary Vessels.*

7. Matsumoto and Birch, *Extraordinary Vessels.*

8. Matsumoto and Birch, *Hara Diagnosis.*

9. *Morohashi's Etymological Dictionary,* quoted in Matsumoto and Birch, *Extraordinary Vessels.*

10. Matsumoto and Birch, *Extraordinary Vessels.*

11. Ibid.

12. H. S. Burr, *Blueprint for Immortality* (London: Neville Spearman Ltd., 1972).

13. Becker, *The Body Electric.*

14. Matsumoto and Birch, *Extraordinary Vessels.*

15. When released into the surrounding tissues, this discharge has a minor local effect. I believe that this is one of the mechanisms responsible for the conversion of matrix material (hyaluronic acid) from its gel state to its sol state—the underlying physiological change that facilitates connective tissue manipulation.

16. Becker showed in his work on frog erythrocytes that physiological tissues can respond to signals as small as one-half of one-billionth (.0000000005) of an ampere. See Becker, *The Body Electric.*

17. Matsumoto and Birch, *Hara Diagnosis.*

18. Becker, *The Body Electric.*

19. Tortora and Anagnostakos, *Principles.*

20. Dr. K. Nakamura, personal communication, 1975.

21. Superconduction is a phenomenon that normally takes place only at temperatures near absolute zero (−273° Celsius). Superconduction reduces the resistance in an electrical circuit to zero, allowing electrically generated activity to go on indefinitely with only a minimal initial input of energy. This is real perpetual motion. Beginning with Albert Szent-Györgyi, it has been theorized that some biological semiconductors such as collagen might support superconduction in living tissues at life-supporting temperatures. See Becker, *The Body Electric.*

BIBLIOGRAPHY

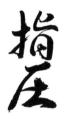

Austin, M. *Acupuncture Therapy*. New York: ASI Pubs., Inc., 1972.

Barral, J. P. and P. Mercier. *Visceral Manipulation*. Seattle: Eastland Press, 1988.

Becker, R. *Cross Currents*. Los Angeles: Jeremy P. Tarcher, 1990.

Becker, R. and A. Marino. *Electromagnetism and Life*. Albany, N.Y.: State University of New York Press, 1982.

Becker, R. and G. Seldon. *The Body Electric: Electromagnetism and the Foundation of Life*. New York: William Morrow, 1985.

Benjamin, B. *Listen To Your Pain*. New York: Penguin Books, 1984.

Bohm, D. *Wholeness and the Implicate Order*. London: Ark Paperbacks, 1980.

Burr, H. S. *Blueprint for Immortality*. London: Neville Spearman Ltd., 1972.

Burr, H. S. and F. S. C. Northrup. "Electro-Dynamic Fields of Life." *Quarterly Review of Biology* 10: 322–33, 1935.

Capra, F. *The Tao of Physics*. New York: Bantam Books, 1976.

Chaitow, L. *Soft-Tissue Manipulation*. Rochester, Vt.: Healing Arts Press, 1987.

Cheng Xinnong, ed. *Chinese Acupuncture and Moxibustion*. Beijing: Foreign Language Press, 1987.

Chia, M. *Chi Nei Tsang*. Huntington, N.Y.: Healing Tao Books, 1990.

Connelly, D. *Traditional Acupuncture: The Law of the Five Elements*. Columbia, Md.: Centre For Traditional Acupuncture, 1979.

Da Free John. *The Eating Gorilla Comes In Peace*. Middletown, Calif.: Dawn Horse Press, 1979.

Dubitsky, C., et al. "Three Paradigms, Five Approaches." *Massage Therapy Journal*, Summer 1991.

Ellis, A., N. Wiseman, and K. Boss. *Fundamentals of Chinese Acupuncture*. Brookline, Mass.: Paradigm Publications, 1988.

Evens, J., *Mind, Body and Electromagmetism*. Longmead, UK.: Element Books, 1981.

Graham, J. *Evening Primrose Oil*. Rochester, Vt.: Healing Arts Press, 1984.

Green, E. and A. Green. *Beyond Biofeedback*. San Francisco: Delacourt Press, 1977.

Haldeman, S. *Modern Developments in the Principles and Practice of Chiropractic*. New York: Appleton-Century-Crofts, 1981.

Harukai, O. *Lao Tze and Chuag Tze, Dao De Jing*. Tokyo: Chuo Koran, 1978.

Jones, L. *Strain and Counterstrain*. Colorado Springs: American Academy of Osteopathy, 1981.

Juhan, D. *Job's Body*. Barrytown, N.Y.: Station Hill Press, 1987.

Kaptchuk, T. *The Web That Has No Weaver*. New York: Congdon and Weed, 1983.

King, R. *Body Mobilization Technique*. Chicago: Chicago School of Massage, 1986.

Kinoshita, H. *Illustration of Acupoints*. Tokyo: Ido-No-Nippon-Sha Press, 1970.

Korr, I. *Spinal Cord as Organizer of Disease Process.* Newark, Ohio: Academy of Applied Osteopathy Yearbook, 1976.

Krieger, D. *Therapeutic Touch.* Englewood Cliffs, N.J.: Prentice-Hall, 1979.

Lee, H. and G. Whincup. *Chinese Massage Therapy: A Handbook of Therapeutic Massage.* Boulder, Colo.: Shambhala, 1983.

Maciocia, G. *Foundations of Chinese Medicine.* Edinburgh: Churchill Livingstone, 1989.

———. *Tongue Diagnosis in Chinese Medicine.* Seattle: Eastland Press, 1987.

Manaka, Y. and I. Urquhart. *Layman's Guide to Acupuncture.* New York: Weatherhill, 1972.

Mann, F. *Acupuncture: The Ancient Chinese Art of Healing and How It Works Scientifically.* New York: Vintage Books, 1979.

Masunaga, S. with W. Ohashi. *Zen Shiatsu.* Tokyo: Japan Press, 1977.

Matsumoto, K. and S. Birch. *Extraordinary Vessels.* Brookline, Mass.: Paradigm Publications, 1986.

———. *Five Elements, Ten Stems.* Brookline, Mass.: Paradigm Publications, 1983.

———. *Hara Diagnosis: Reflections on the Sea.* Brookline, Mass.: Paradigm Publications, 1988.

Meagher, J. and P. Boughton. *Sportsmassage.* Garden City, N.J.: Doubleday, 1980.

Mizutani, J. "A Brief History." *Shiatsu Therapy of Ontario Newsletter,* September 1991.

Moor, F. et al. *Manual of Hydrotherapy and Massage.* Mountain View, Calif.: Pacific Press, 1964.

Nakagawa, K. "Magnetic Field Deficiency Syndrome and Magnetic Treatment." *Japan Medical Journal* No. 2745, December 4, 1976.

Namikoshi, T. *The Complete Book of Shiatsu Therapy.* Tokyo: Japan Publishers, 1981.

Netter, F. *Atlas of Human Anatomy.* Summit, N.J.: Ciba-Geigy, 1989.

O'Connor, J. and D. Bensky. *Acupuncture: A Comprehensive Text.* Seattle: Eastland Press, 1981.

Palmer, D. "On-Site Massage: Responding to the Mainstream." *Massage Therapy Journal,* vol. 11, no. 1, Winter 1987.

Pearson, D. and S. Shaw. *Life Extension.* New York: Warner Books, 1982.

Pelletier, K. *Mind as Healer, Mind as Slayer.* New York: Delta Press, 1977.

Phaigh, R and P. Perry. *Athletic Massage.* New York: Simon and Schuster, 1984.

Phipps, Toshiko. "History of Shiatsu." *American Shiatsu Association Newsletter,* Winter 1986.

Requena, Y. *Terrains and Pathology in Acupuncture.* Brookline, Mass.: Paradigm Publications, 1986.

Rolf, I. *Integration of Human Structures.* Santa Monica, Calif.: Landman Publishers, 1977.

Ross, J. *Zang Fu: The Organ Systems of Traditional Chinese Medicine,* 2nd ed. Edinburgh: Churchill Livingstone, 1985.

Seem, M. *Bodymind Energetics.* Rochester, Vt.: Healing Arts Press, 1988.

Selye, H. *The Stress of Life.* New York: McGraw Hill, 1976.

Serizawa, K. *Tsubo: Vital Points for Oriental Therapy.* Tokyo: Japan Publishers, 1976.

Sohn, T. *Amma: The Ancient Art of Oriental Healing.* Rochester, Vt.: Healing Arts Press, 1989.

Sun Chengnan, ed. *Chinese Bodywork: A Complete Manual of Chinese Therapeutic Massage.* Berkely, Calif.: Pacific View Press, 1993.

Sun Simiao. *Thousand Ducat Prescriptions,* 3rd ed. Taiwan: National Chinese Medical Herbal Research Center Publishing Co., 1980.

Taber's Cyclopedic Medical Dictionary, 14th ed. Philadelphia: F. A. Davis, 1981.

Tappan, F. *Healing Massage Techniques.* New York: Appleton & Lange, 1987.

Toguchi, M. and F. Warren. *Complete Guide to Acupuncture/Acupressure.* New York: Gramercy, 1985.

Tortora, G. and N. Anagnostakos. *Principles of Anatomy and Physiology,* 4th ed. New York: Harper and Row, 1984.

Upledger, J. and J. Vredevoogd. *Craniosacral Therapy.* Seattle: Eastland Press, 1983.

Walford, R. *Maximum Life Span.* New York: W. W. Norton, 1983.

Wittlinger, H. *Textbook of Dr. Vodder's Manual Lymph Drainage.* Vol. 1: Basic course. 5th ed. Heidelberg, Ger.: Carl F. Haug, 1995.

Yamamoto, S. *Barefoot Shiatsu.* Tokyo: Japan Publishers, 1979.

Zhen, Li Shi. *Pulse Diagnosis.* Brookline, Mass.: Paradigm Publications, 1985.

INDEX

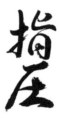

Notes are indexed by page, chapter, and note number thus: 243 n. 6.1